BF 637 .C6 P64 1996

Posthuma, Barbara W., 1931-

Coun Small groups in counseling
and therapy

JUN 6 1998			
SEP 6 1998			

DEMCO 38-297

Related Titles of Interest

**Group Design and Leadership: Strategies for Creating
  Successful Common Theme Groups**
Henry B. Andrews
ISBN: 0-205-16197-9

**The Professional Counselor: A Process Guide
  to Helping, Second Edition**
J. Sherilyn Cormier and Harold Hackney
ISBN: 0-205-14156-0

**Foundations and Applications of Group
  Psychotherapy: A Sphere of Influence**
Mark F. Ettin
ISBN: 0-205-13508-0

**Joining Together: Group Theory and Group Skills,
  Fifth Edition**
David W. Johnson and Frank P. Johnson
ISBN: 0-205-15846-3

Foundations of Therapeutic Interviewing
John Sommers-Flanagan and Rita Sommers-Flanagan
ISBN: 0-205-14063-7

SECOND EDITION

Small Groups in Counseling and Therapy

Process and Leadership

Barbara W. Posthuma

University of Western Ontario

Allyn and Bacon

Boston   London   Toronto   Sydney   Tokyo   Singapore

Allyn & Bacon
A Simon & Schuster Company
Needham Heights, Massachusetts 02194

The first edition of this book was published under the title *Small
Groups in Therapy Settings: Process and Leadership,* copyright © 1989
by Barbara Posthuma.

Library of Congress Cataloging-in-Publication Data

Posthuma, Barbara W., date-
    Small groups in counseling and therapy: process and leadership /
Barbara W. Posthuma.—2nd ed.
        p.   cm.
    Includes bibliographical references and index.
    ISBN 0-205-16169-3
    1. Group counseling.   2. Group psychotherapy.   1. Title.
BF637.C6P64   1996
158'.35—dc20
                                                    95-15081
                                                    CIP

Printed in the United States of America
10   9   8   7   6   5   4   3   99   98   97   96

*To
Kristy and Kerry,
my original group*

Contents

Preface

The purpose of writing the first edition of this book still holds for this second edition: to produce a suitable textbook for educators who teach group dynamics. My methods of teaching the concepts and practical skills necessary for effective small group leadership have remained both didactic and experiential. It is hoped that this revised edition retains both these styles of presentation.

The original book was targeted specifically to my own profession— occupational therapy. Many readers felt this focus was too limiting, however, so an effort has been made to broaden the context. It is hoped that this new edition retains the flavor that made the original attractive to occupational therapists while expanding the contextual content to appeal to counselors, educators, nurses, social workers, therapists, and other group practitioners. To work effectively with small groups, all professionals need the same basic conceptual knowledge about group process, group development, and leadership. *Small Groups in Counseling and Therapy* attempts to meet these general and universal needs.

Based on solicited and unsolicited feedback as well as suggestions from both colleagues and students, the chronology of the content has been reorganized. It is felt that this new flow follows a more orderly or "first things first" approach to the study of small groups. Because of the proliferation of self-help groups in communities everywhere, a chapter dealing with this phenomenon has been added. At some time during the professional careers of all health, education, and social practitioners there will be a point of involvement in or a need for information regarding self-help groups.

In an effort to avoid the awkward referent *he/she,* the format of using the female pronoun in all instances to refer to the group leader and the male pronoun to refer to group members is continued in this edition. The information contained in the appendices, while somewhat changed, is included to demonstrate how several group sessions can be organized around a single theme. The activities for each session are suggested and described to give the novice leader some format ideas as well as specific ideas for immediate use.

Acknowledgments

I would like to take this opportunity to acknowledge the helpful and constructive comments of the four reviewers of the first edition. They are Nancy Blake, Towson State University; Thomas Caulfield, Canisius College; Elizabeth Holloway, University of Wisconsin; and Janet Falk-Kessler, Columbia University. Many of their suggestions have been incorporated into this second edition.

While the process of revision was primarily a singular endeavor, my acknowledgments for support with the original text, although not reiterated here, still stand. I wish to thank Susan Weeks and Lynne Helwig for their computer expertise and helpful skills in manipulating the manuscript. Most of all I want to thank my husband Allan Sexton for his continuing support and understanding while I rewrote "the book."

B.W.P.

About the Author

Barbara Posthuma has been a Professor at the University of Western Ontario in the Department of Occupational Therapy since 1973. During that time she has published many manuscripts in a variety of professional refereed journals as well as the first edition of this book. She has taught several courses in the area of mental health including courses on communication, group dynamics, assessment, and interviewing. Barbara has given many presentations on small groups, including keynote addresses at conferences, and workshops at a variety of venues in Canada, the United States, New Zealand, Australia, Portugal, and Germany. She has also been involved in the World Federation of Occupational Therapists since 1982 and has served as Honorary Secretary since 1986. Barbara has two daughters who live in Vancouver, British Columbia, while she and her husband, Allan Sexton, live in London, Ontario, Canada.

The road to wisdom? Well it's plain
and simple to express:
Err
And err
And err again
But less
And less
And less

— PIET HEIN

Small Groups in Counseling and Therapy

Chapter 1

The Small Group in Counseling and Therapy

*We must conclude that the
psychology of groups is the oldest
human psychology.*
— SIGMUND FREUD

From the beginning of time people congregated in groups to ensure their survival, development, and evolution. The knowledge that there was safety in numbers was a motivating factor in the earliest gatherings of people. Other factors that drew people together were spiritual in nature as groups of people congregated to worship, celebrate, and perform ritual dances. These original groups were formed naturally either by shared ancestry, mutual need, or common belief. In noting these beginnings Rudestam (1982) states: "Despite the pervasiveness of such groups throughout history, the connections between them and the deliberate use of group process to foster personality change in the twentieth century have not been made explicit" (p 1). Although early theorists did not directly connect or address the behavior of individuals in groups in relation to therapeutic possibilities, sociologists and social psychologists did actively begin to raise questions and investigate the nuances of collective behavior late in the nineteenth century (Hare, 1992).

J. R. and L. M. Gibb (1978) observed that "groups form the fabric of the society in which we live" (p. 106) and early investigations focused primarily on examining the effects of social influences on the behavior of individuals. One such exploration, credited to psychologist Norman Triplett in 1887, demonstrated that a cyclist's performance could be significantly improved if he or she was accompanied or paced by another rider (Bonner, 1959; Rudestam, 1982). Other researchers of this time studied the effect of working alone versus working in groups, pertaining to the performance of children

1

in school, the influence of a group on thought processes, and the effect of competition on performance (Bonner, 1959). F. H. Allport, whose work is frequently documented in the early literature on groups, found that individuals working in a group produced more verbal associations and presented such associations with greater speed than did individuals working alone (Allport, 1920).

Later investigators (Comrey & Staats, 1955; Goldman, 1965) went on to compare individual and group performance using different combinations of individuals with varying initial ability. They found that the improved performance demonstrated by working in a dyad or a group was dependent on the initial ability levels of the individuals who were in combination.

In their review of the literature, Rosenbaum and Berger (1975) conclude that the primary early researchers noted for investigating small group phenomena were: Charles H. Cooley, who first defined the concept of "the primary group" as the "face to face" group primarily involved with "intimate cooperation"; Gustave Le Bon, who first described the group as a "collective entity—a distinct being"; and George Herbert Mead whose work, along with that of Cooley, was "of prime significance in the early history of group dynamics" (p. 13).

From these early explorations into the forces affecting individuals as they participated in groups evolved the use of groups as vehicles to promote change. One of the first practitioners credited with using this approach was Joseph Pratt, a Boston internist. Although Pratt originally used groups to save time in educating and supporting patients suffering from tuberculosis, he later became aware of the therapeutic value of the format, in particular the interactions among members of such groups. His work is acknowledged as an important forerunner to present-day psychotherapy (Scheidlinger & Schamess, 1992).

Recognized as being the "founder of the study of modern group dynamics" (Luft, 1984, p. 8), social psychologist Kurt Lewin's work as a theorist and researcher in the investigation of group dynamics had a significant impact on the use of groups as agents for change (Smith, 1980a). The work of Lewin and his associates is credited with having a direct bearing on the invention of the T-group (training group), from which evolved the encounter and sensitivity groups of the 1960s and 1970s. The widespread interest in these groups grew, in part, from the increased feelings of alienation that were experienced by an expanding portion of an increasingly mobile society (Scheidlinger & Schamess, 1992). Caring, trust, and the process of feedback, such as the sharing of perceptions both among members and with the leader, were encouraged in these groups. Emphasis was put on the importance of discussing events and behaviors happening in the "here-and-now" in the group.

Most reviews of the historical development of group work methods mark World War II as being a catalyst to increased interest and innovation in the use of groups (Rosenbaum, 1976; Scheidlinger & Schamess, 1992; Smith,

1980b). The shortage of trained therapists and the need to treat an increasing number of veterans precipitated a greater use of groups for therapy. Around this time the work of J. L. Moreno, who is best remembered as the founder of psychodrama, was gaining much recognition. He is credited with organizing the first society of group therapists, coining the term "group psychotherapy," and introducing the first professional journal on group therapy (Blatner, 1989). The basic premise of Moreno's *psychodrama* was an action technique to bring about both mental and emotional catharsis for the purpose of relieving tension. Although intense and extensive training is required to qualify as a certified director of psychodrama, several of the individual techniques can be learned and effectively used by leaders of small groups. Indeed, many explorative and spontaneous group leaders have intuitively used techniques such as role reversal and mirroring as part of role-playing sessions without thought of any connection to classic psychodrama.

Two trends emerged from 1932 to the 1960s in the years known as the "developmental period" of group psychotherapy (Shapiro, 1978). The first trend was the spreading application of the group method in the treatment of a wider variety of patient populations and the second was the use of groups for purposes of personal growth and preservation. The latter trend culminated in the 1960s (Ramey, 1992) when there was "a group for everyone and everyone was in a group" (Gladding, 1991, p. 9). One would be remiss to leave even such a brief overview of the developmental period without noting the emergence of Alcoholics Anonymous. The founding of this movement in the late 1930s evolved from the awareness of the potency of individuals meeting together and interacting in a supportive way to produce change. This organization, which has a well-recorded success rate in helping alcoholics attain and maintain sobriety, is based on individuals coming together in groups for the shared experiences of disclosing, talking, listening, supporting, and learning (Alcoholics Anonymous World Service, 1984). Since then other self-help groups focusing on a myriad of specific problems have evolved and are discussed in depth in Chapter 14.

ADVANTAGES OF GROUPS

Although early group leaders, trained and entrenched in the one-to-one method of psychotherapy, tended to carry this format into the group setting (Ormont, 1992), by the 1950s "group therapy was emerging as an important modality" (Dusay & Dusay, 1989, p. 412). This new modality was found to enable clients to develop feelings of belonging and awareness of others, to increase socialization skills, to experience increased self-confidence, and to offer opportunities for the exchange of ideas (Nelson, Mackenthun, Bloesch, Milan, Unrein, & Hill, 1956). Shannon and Snortum (1965) observed at the time that "by working in a group of limited size, the patient could be provided with a more closely supervised opportunity for practicing rudimentary social skills and receive needed feedback from actual experience, thereby discovering that he is capable of handling social situations that formerly prompted his withdrawal" (p. 345). Following this, although research into the effectiveness of groups was sporadic and limited (Gladding, 1991), investigations carried out by sociologists, psychologists, psychiatrists, and other professionals into the value of small groups "recognized the group's curative powers and sought to use them to achieve therapeutic goals" (Howe & Schwartzberg, 1986, p. 52).

Since then groups have proliferated with great vigor and variety among most of the helping professions. It is difficult, and perhaps not wise, to generalize, but it seems safe to say that groups have been effective in short-term psychiatric settings (Bradlee, 1984; McLees, Margo, Waterman, & Beeber, 1992; Prazoff, Joyce & Azim, 1986), long-term psychiatric settings (Waldinger, 1990; Wolf, 1975), counseling for special populations (Corey & Corey, 1992; Corey, 1990), and with the chronically physically ill (Buchanan, 1978; Levine, 1979). Garland (1992) notes a renewed popularity of groups in the 1990s that deal with issues such as violence, sexual abuse, lawbreaking, addictions, phobias, and eating disorders. As leaders move into the twenty-first century, speculation is that therapists and counselors alike will need to be competent in leading counseling groups, prevention groups, community development teams, as well as psychotherapy groups (Conyne, Harvill, Morganett, Morran, & Hulse-Killacky, 1990).

THERAPEUTIC AND COUNSELING GROUPS

The main purpose of all counseling and therapeutic endeavors is to bring about change. When a person joins a counseling group, it is usually to learn new ways of being, interrelating, and interacting. In a therapeutic small group the specific goals for each member can be varied but would include the expectation that change will occur (Levine, 1979). In both types of groups it is expected that members will become more functional and less distressed. Often groups are called by names that indicate their purpose. For example, both therapists and counselors run communication groups, assertiveness groups, life-skills groups, and decision-making groups. The general goals of these respective groups are to improve communication skills, to increase assertiveness, to provide experience in life-skills, and to allow experience in a decision-making process.

If the theme of the group is self-awareness, then one goal for the group members would be to become more aware of various aspects of themselves—of how they behave in different situations, how they react to certain stimuli, and how others react and behave in return. A second goal would be for the members to use this new awareness to gain a better understanding of themselves and, based on this understanding, to effect some change in their behavior directed at achieving or eliciting more productive outcomes.

Immediately the question arises, "What happens in groups that enable members to change?" Or, as Kottler (1983) asks, "What is this magic that cures people of their suffering?" (p. 51). Perhaps the magic in part is based on the phenomenon described by Kurt Lewin who is credited with the observation that "it is usually easier to change individuals formed into a group than to change any one of them separately" (Rosenbaum & Berger, 1975, p. 16). In commenting on the process and the helpful aspects of self-help groups Lieberman (1990a) says: "The group member is almost inevitably confronted with pressure from others to change behaviors and views" (p. 260). Although a person does not experience the same one-to-one attention in a group as she or he would receive during individual counseling or therapy there are other factors that contribute to the success of groups as a therapeutic modality. Rudestam (1982) discusses five elements that he considers to be advantages of using groups to facilitate bringing about change.

First, Rudestam likens a group to a "miniature society" where members can lose their feelings of alienation and, temporarily at least, experience feelings of belonging, thus meeting one of the basic needs of humankind (Maslow, 1968). Within the group setting members can experience everyday life situations such as peer pressure, social influence, and the need to conform. In this microcosm of society members can relate their behavior in the group to their behavior in social groups outside the group. When these experiences occur in a learning environment, such as a group, then the changes that occur are usually transferable to the outside world (Posthuma, 1972; Waldinger, 1990).

The second element in favor of the group treatment setting is the opportunity to be among others with whom common problems can be shared. It offers the chance to learn new skills and behaviors in a supportive environment. Through group interaction one can receive feedback and caring, experience trust and acceptance, and learn new ways of relating to others. Because most groups are comprised of a cross section of members of society at large, this affords each group member opportunities to cope with give-and-take situations similar to those existing in the world outside. In one-to-one therapy the client experiences only one other point of view and one source of feedback, that of the therapist. While such viewpoints and feedback may be valid, they are limited in breadth and experience by virtue of coming from only one person (Ferencik, 1992). In a group the client may experience several points of view and varied feedback (Ormont, 1992), as shown in Figure 1–1, all of which may be presented in different ways. By evaluating this assortment of information, the group member is able to select what he feels could be of personal value and assistance.

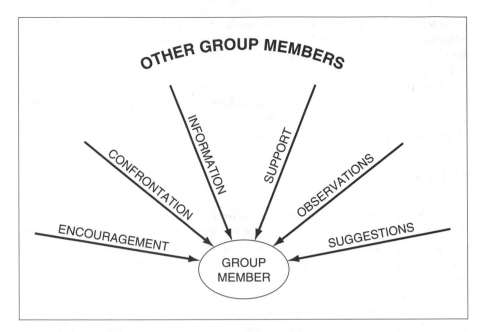

Figure 1–1. Sample of varied feedback available to each group member.

Hopefully, because of this mixture, group members will get a broader view of themselves and become more aware of the more subtle nuances of their behavior. Also, the integration of information is likely to produce a combination of supportive and confrontive messages that can soften any good–bad or right–wrong dichotomies. The more supportive feedback serves as a sort of cushion for the more confrontive. In essence this multifeedback situation creates an environment in which members are more receptive and feel less need to be defensive and block out negative feedback (Campbell, 1992). They are more apt to listen, to take in, and to consider what they hear and hence benefit from the process. Conversely, it is also true that there is strength in numbers. It is easier to disregard feedback that comes from one source only with a "what-does-he-know?" attitude. However, it is close to impossible to ignore feedback from five or more persons if they share the same perceptions and are all giving the same messages or information.

Third, the individual is able to observe the problems, struggles, behaviors, interaction styles, and coping mechanisms of the others in the group. He is then able to use this information as a yardstick for comparing his own behaviors. From this a group member can assess his own abilities and disabilities and consider possibilities for personal change.

Closely linked to the third advantage is the fourth, which is the facilitation of the individual growth process. The support of the group can be an enhancing factor in self-exploration and introspection (Lieberman, 1990b; Posthuma & Posthuma, 1972). Feeling, caring, and respect from others can go a long way in promoting the self-confidence necessary to attempt new and different ways of behaving.

The final advantage of the group format for both counseling and therapy is the obvious one of economics. Having several clients meet together with a group leader rather than meeting individually with a therapist or counselor saves time and money (Davies & Gavin, 1994).

TERMINOLOGY

Before going further a clarification of terminology is in order. In any discussion of small groups the terms *group dynamics* and *group process* are frequently used. Comments such as "There were some powerful dynamics in that group" or "The process in the group today was really interesting" are often made by group leaders or observers of small group sessions. So what do these terms mean? While noting that the term *group dynamics* can refer to a field of study and a body of knowledge, Jacobs, Harvill, and Masson (1988) concisely define group dynamics in its most basic sense as "the forces that are operating in a group" (p. 23). These forces include "nonverbal behaviors, communication patterns, levels of participation, expression of feelings, and resistances and avoidances" (Brown, 1992, p. 20). The term *group process,* Fried (1972) says, should be used specifically to refer to the patterns of interactions that develop among members at various times during a group. Gladding (1991) says that group dynamics lead to group processes whereas Gillette and McCollom (1990) include "distinct processes" in their definition of group dynamics. It seems that this confusion over terms is inevitable because the complex forces and the interactions are all occurring simultaneously and the forces may well affect the interactions and, conversely, the interactions among the members may alter and affect the forces. Because of this concurrent, intimate, and ongoing relationship between the two, for the purposes of this book the two terms will be used interchangeably to mean the same thing: everything and anything that is happening in a group, whether the occurrence is seen to be overt or covert.

HOW CHANGE OCCURS

Change leads people into the realm of the unknown and the realization of this can be frightening. There are no certainties with change, and undefined future experiences and situations create resistance to change in everyone. People invest a great deal of energy in preserving the status quo as a defense against change. People often say, "That's the way I am," as a means of ending any further discussion of behaviors or alternatives.

There are no guarantees that change will make things better for a person or that others will agree on what constitutes "better." When a person does change some aspect of his way of "being" in the world, the change in behavior will not necessarily be seen as beneficial by all who are close to him (Posthuma & Posthuma, 1973). For example, the increasing conflict and confusion between the sexes, which are in part brought about by social changes as women take on more traditionally male roles in the workplace and expect men to take on more traditionally female tasks in the home, are frequently discussed in the popular literature (Johnson, 1994).

The need for change comes when people find some aspect of their lives unbearable, or when those close to them find aspects of their behavior unacceptable (Hansen, Warner, & Smith, 1980). Conditions, such as loneliness, a poor relationship, lack of a job, drinking, fears, or losses, may be perceived as problems. Kanfer and Goldstein (1986) state that generally psychological problems are related to difficulties in relationships, in attitudes toward the self, or in perceptions of the environment. They cite four characteristics (presented here in part) that they believe indicate evidence of the presence of a psychological problem.

1. The person experiences discomfort, worry, or fears that are not easily remedied by some action that can be performed without assistance.
2. The person shows a behavioral deficiency or excessively engages in some behavior that is assessed by himself or herself or others to interfere with normal functioning.
3. The person engages in activities that are objectionable to those around him and that lead to negative consequences either personally or for others.
4. The person shows behavioral deviations that result in severe social sanctions by those in the immediate environment (p. 8).

The beginning of the change process is marked by the recognition that something must be altered. At this point the individual may try to make changes by himself, or he may turn to family members or friends. The person may seek out a counselor/therapist or join a counseling/therapeutic group. Whatever avenue he chooses through which to find help, the change process that ensues tends to be similar. In relationships with others he finds individuals, therapists, counselors, or group members who are accepting and who listen to his thoughts and feelings. Within this environment of acceptance and positive regard he is able to recognize and realize the existence of previously denied feelings and behaviors (Raskin & Rogers, 1989). This enables the client to reorganize his self-perceptions in ways that allow him to gradually accept himself and to see himself as a person of worth and even one worthy of further enhancement.

Yalom (1985) discusses "therapeutic factors" (originally called "curative factors") which he says operate in all types of therapy groups, with different factors being emphasized in any given group depending on the goals and composition of the group and the approach that is being used. It is also true that in some situations clients must deal with certain factors before they can benefit from others (Bonney, Randall, & Cleveland, 1986). Other authors have identified "helping factors" (Schulz, 1993; Schwartzberg, 1993) in support groups that appear similar in many respects to Yalom's therapeutic factors.

Yalom notes that many of the factors are interdependent and that some factors represent conditions for change while others are actually mechanisms of change. Yalom's factors have been extensively cited and investigated, including recent research that explored the timing of testing as being a determinant of which factors group members would consider to be the most effective change agents. MacKenzie (1987) established that outcome measures evaluating the usefulness of the therapeutic factors, when taken retrospectively, differed from results obtained while members were still active in the group. Descriptions of the ten primary categories of therapeutic factors follow (Yalom, 1985).

1. *Imparting of Information.* The type of information imparted in groups will depend on the type of group, the leader, and the members. Included may be advice, suggestions, guidance, interpretations, or didactic instruction about a certain theoretical approach such as transactional analysis or cognitive restructuring. In task groups such as assertiveness training, life skills, or goal setting, it is likely that the leader will give information and instructions to the members before commencing the activity. In using a didactic approach, one must be careful that the group does not become essentially a "class" and hence foster a dependence on the leader to "tell us what to do." This caution is basically supported by the work of Block and Crouch (1985) who found guidance to be one of the least helpful therapeutic factors. In a self-help group for persons suffering from asthma, however, Llewelyn and Haslett (1986) found that the "guidance" factor was the most helpful. Members appeared to appreciate the opportunity to learn more about their condition from both professionals and their peers. In a study with clients in a psychiatric day treatment center Falk-Kessler, Momich, and Perel (1991) found that whereas group leaders found guidance to be valuable the group members did not.

2. *Installation of Hope.* It is crucial that members see the group as a helpful–hopeful treatment method. Many groups are open, so new members are being accepted as others approach discharge. This process offers the opportunity for those members who have gained and improved from the group experience to share their experiences with the newer members. If Joe can say, "When I first came into this group I was scared and didn't think I had anything worthwhile to say, so I was pretty quiet. But now I think I talk as much as anyone," then this can give encouragement and hope to a timid, withdrawn member that he too may be able to reach that point. Yalom (1985) actually encourages leaders to "exploit" this factor by pointing out changes and improvements that members have made as a means of offering hope to others.

3. *Universality.* Each group member is different, having his very own set of unique problems. Members often believe that no one else could possibly have problems that are as bad as theirs. However, as members begin to talk in the group and as the "bad" problems are shared, members come to experience a join-the-club feeling. As members listen to disclosures made by other clients, they sense a similarity of concerns and issues. This helps them put their own problems into perspective and tends to alleviate feelings of aloneness which dissolves the feeling of "I am the only one." In a study of three self-help groups, Lieberman (1983) reports that *universality*—the feeling of being with others who share the same problems—was the experience the members valued the most. In losing their feelings of uniqueness members came to perceive their thoughts and feelings not as being aberrant and unusual but as being quite common among those with similar problems. While this dispelling of feelings of isolation is therapeutic in itself, it also facilitates a feeling of unity among the members that is the very foundation for a successful group.

4. *Altruism.* One of the basic premises of therapeutic groups is that the members will help each other. The trust and cohesion that evolve in groups supply fertile ground for patients to give feedback, reassurance, suggestions, and support to one another. Since many individuals who are members of counseling or therapy groups suffer from low self-esteem, this process of being able to help others can be a very ego-strengthening experience. It is often the group members, rather than the leader, who offer support and caring and point out one another's strengths and assets.

5. *Family Reenactment.* Although other researchers (Block, Crouch, & Reibstein, 1981; MacDevitt & Sanislow, 1987) have found family reenactment to be one of the least helpful factors, Yalom (1985) recognized the familial aspects of a therapeutic group as being useful. Many patients will have had unsatisfactory, if not traumatic, family experiences. Reporting on a study involving a group of incest victims, Bonney, Randall, and Cleveland (1986) found that the members placed a heavy emphasis on gaining genetic insight through self-understanding and family reenactment. As well as gaining understanding of the past, being in a group gives members the opportunity to experience what can be felt as a caring family environment. Within this group "family" they can discuss and perhaps resolve issues from their primary family such as parent–child conflicts and sibling rivalries. Borrowing from their professional colleagues, the psychodramatists, group leaders often use role-playing in their groups to re-create family situations so that members can learn new ways of relating and interacting within their own families.

6. *Development of Socializing Techniques.* The assessment and development of social skills has long been of prime interest to counselors and therapists alike. Social skills are prerequisites for most people to function adequately in their life roles. Most of our clients, however, experience difficulties in one if not several of their life roles and their problems can, in part, be attributed to poor social skills. The process of feedback, mentioned earlier, affords the opportunity to learn about one's maladaptive social behavior. For individuals who lack close personal relationships in their lives, the group is often the first time they have had an opportunity to give and receive personal feedback. Role-playing, a technique often used in groups, can be used successfully both in increasing awareness of and in teaching social skills. This technique is discussed more fully in Chapter 13.

7. *Imitative Behaviour.* In any group each participant has the opportunity to observe, at close hand and in an interactive manner, the behaviors of all the other participants. Through such observations they become aware of which behaviors evoke positive and negative responses from the other members. By imitating or "trying on" these behaviors they too can evoke such responses. Behaviors that receive a positive reaction from others are usually repeated and hence new learning can occur. Some members may imitate certain behaviors of the leaders or other members only to later discard them, deciding the "fit" is not comfortable. This too is learning. Of course there can also be the member who imitates the "bad" person in the group in order to receive the same degree of attention, even if it is negative attention.

8. *Interpersonal Learning.* No one goes through life alone. Rudestam (1982) says, "Life is primarily a social event" (p. 6). A person may feel lonely and alienated or be considered a loner but the demands of daily existence, be they work or play, tend to involve one in relating to others. Because a group is considered a miniature society (Rudestam, 1982) or a microcosm of reality (Ormont, 1992) it presents similar demands. Initially, members of a group, or a new member in an ongoing group, may monitor and control how they behave. However, it is anticipated that eventually each person will relax and come to behave as he normally does in his own social environment. Each person will affect the other members of the group in much the same way as he affects people he has contact with in the greater society. By virtue of the purpose and the process of a therapeutic group, members will receive feedback on their "way of being" and from these reactions and responses they have the opportunity to learn how they affect others. Spurred by this feedback, and the support and encouragement of the group, they can, it is hoped, go on to learn more productive ways of interacting. The trust and caring that develops in a group creates a safer environment for experimentation and for trying out new ways of relating than does the environment of society at large.

In an assessment of Yalom's therapeutic factors, Lewis (1987) states a case for the importance of interactions between people in the process of bringing about change. He believes that a person can interact with another in a way to elicit a desired response. He refers to these as "complementary responses" and because they are new and different from the person's usual response style they constitute a change. Positive reactions to the new interactive style serves as a reward and reinforcer for continuance of the changed behavior. Lewis's point is in keeping with the belief that people often live up (or down) to perceived expectations.

9. *Cohesion.* The concept of cohesion is central to any discussion of the elements contributing to the successful functioning of groups. This concept has been accorded many definitions but they all have a common theme. Words such as "unity," "bonded," "we-ness," "cemented," and "loyalty" are all used to describe a state of cohesion in a group. Yalom (1985) also notes that it is not a static state, but rather the degree of cohesiveness present in a group fluctuates over time and circumstance. He goes on to point out that cohesion in and of itself does not have therapeutic properties but is an important determinant that effective therapy is occurring. It is during periods when a group is experiencing a feeling of unity or togetherness that members are more apt to contribute, take risks, interact, and be productive (Evans & Dion, 1991).

Mullen (1992) suggests that "cohesion's easy occurrence, in so many disparate group therapies, is less a result of therapist skill than of innate patient capacity" (p. 460). Members who are attracted to the group, feel accepted, and experience a sense of belonging are more apt to express and explore themselves, relate more meaningfully, be more tolerant of conflict, and attend regularly (Dimock, 1985a). In two separate studies evaluating the merits of Yalom's therapeutic factors in task groups, the results indicated that cohesion was found to be the most valued factor by the group members (Falk-Kessler, Momich, & Perel, 1990; Webster & Schwartzberg, 1992).

10. *Catharsis.* Catharsis refers to the expression of strong emotions and usually emotions that have not been expressed previously. Although this factor was described as "low prestige but irrepressible" in Yalom's early work, by 1985 he found catharsis to be one of the four factors valued most highly by a variety of outpatients in eight different investigations. In other research it emerged as being *the* most important factor (Lieberman & Videka-Sherman, 1986; Long & Cope, 1980; MacDevitt & Sanislow, 1987).

Taken in the perspective of today's highly pressured society, this high ranking can be seen to make a lot of sense. Many of us live our lives by controlling our emotions and not showing the world how we really feel. To display emotions, especially in public, is generally considered poor form and a sign of weakness. Indeed, boys especially are frequently admonished to hide their feelings and "be a big boy" or "be a man." Therefore it is not surprising that when these restrictions and attitudes are not present, as in a group, individuals experience a sense of freedom and release from tension. These good feelings come from being allowed and even encouraged to "get it off our chest" while still feeling respect and acceptance.

Moreno (1957) spoke of the healing effect of catharsis and Janov (1972) of expunging "primal" pain through catharsis. A study by Lieberman, Yalom, and Miles (1973) pointed out that catharsis per se was not necessarily curative; but when coupled with a form of cognitive learning, it could produce a positive outcome. Behaviors that are considered to be cathartic in nature and therapeutic in outcome are the expression of feelings about the self or the expression of positive or negative feelings to others. Such expressions need not always be intense or explosive to be cathartic. The act of a group member mildly expressing how he is feeling can be a new and freeing event for that individual and can frequently evoke similar output from others.

Yalom's ten therapeutic factors endorse the belief that groups are a valuable modality in facilitating change. The need for change is often precipitated by one of the many transitions that people face in a society of "temporary structure" (Seashore, 1974). Temporariness is evident in the high divorce rate, increased geographic relocations, broken families, career changes, and shortened careers. Some people manage to adjust and functionally survive the stresses in their lives, while others, unable to cope, retreat with their problems into a world of varying degrees of dysfunction. Groups have been utilized and found to be of significant help by both types of persons. For those who are adapting and adjusting, groups have served to enhance their coping skills. For the others, groups are therapeutic in nature and remedial in intent (Smith, Wood, & Smale, 1980). While all groups are oriented toward change, some focus primarily on intrapsychic and intrapersonal change, whereas others focus on effecting change in interpersonal skills and relationships.

SUMMARY

The concept of people living and working together is as old as time itself. Although various congregations of people may have been at war or in conflict with each other, the individuals within each group were held together by common purposes and feelings of safety and belonging.

Similar basic aspects pull people together today. People join groups because they like the others in the group, they like the activity or purpose of the group, they want to experience feelings of belonging, or they find they can only accomplish a personal goal by participating with others (e.g., to be a leader, help a cause, or take part in an activity). It can be useful for group leaders to keep these basic motives in mind when organizing and trying to meet the needs of the members in their groups.

Participating in a group can be a powerful social experience, as much as it can be motivating, enlightening, and emotional. As various professionals noted these social effects on individuals who were involved in groups, the professionals became more and more aware of the significance of group interaction. Generally, groups have come to be seen as valuable because they allow members opportunities to have the following positive experiences:

1. A sense of belonging
2. Sharing common problems
3. Observing behaviors and consequences of behaviors in others
4. Support during self-exploration and change

Therapeutically, groups are useful because they bring people together to work on their individual problems in concert. The therapeutic factors that occur when individuals are interacting are:

1. Sharing information
2. Gaining hope
3. Sharing problems
4. Helping one another
5. Experiencing the group as a family
6. Developing social skills
7. Imitating behaviors of others
8. Learning and trying out new behaviors
9. Experiencing cohesion with others
10. Expressing emotions

Groups have great supportive value for persons with minor or severe problems, with or without insight, and in formal or informal settings. The use of groups can also solve certain financial problems by reducing the cost of treatment, because several persons can work together at the same time with one counselor or therapist.

Chapter 2

Group Development

I am not now that which I have been.
— LORD BYRON

Before the meaning of a group's developmental process can be grasped it is necessary to understand the structure of groups and how a group is conceptualized in the overall scheme of things. The perspective chosen from which to examine a group is that of the group as a system. It is hoped that the following brief discussion of a group from this framework will emphasize the many intricacies and complexities inherent in any group. After establishing a group as a many-faceted entity, the rest of the chapter is devoted to the presentation of two models of group development.

Discrepancies existed among the pioneering researchers in how they viewed and described the phenomenon called a *group.* There were those who believed that a group is the sum of its parts: a collective of individual persons participating together. In other words, even though the persons participate in a group, they in essence remain individuals and do not form a whole (Bonner, 1959).

Others believed that although a group is a collection of individuals, their individuality is affected by virtue of the fact that they come together as a group. By coming together, the group of individuals no longer is the sum of its parts, but is a complete entity in and of itself. Accepting the premise that there is some truth in each of these views of a group, one of individuality and one of wholeness, it would then follow that group members can swing back and forth between the two. This being the case, Douglas (1991) notes that a group works best when neither position overwhelms the other.

Others argue that while individual members in a group do not remain as such nor do they lose themselves entirely to the group, what they do in fact is enter into mutual relationships with others and these relationships form a pattern of interacting persons (Tziner & Eden, 1985). It is this pattern of mutuality, known as a group, that is examined here.

THE GROUP AS A SYSTEM

Closely related to the idea of mutuality is the definition of a *system* set forth by Hall and Fagen (1968). They state: "A system is a set of *objects* together with *relationships* between the objects and between their *attributes* (p. 81 [italics added])". Hall and Fagen go on to explain that the *objects* of a system are considered to be the "parts or components" that are "unlimited in variety." The *attributes* are described as the "properties of the objects" and the *relationships* are what "tie the system together." A system, then, is made up of a variety of parts each of which also has properties and all of which are tied together by relationships.

Applying Hall and Fagen's definition to a group, the following identifications can be made. The "parts" are perceived as the group members, the "properties" as the personalities of the members, and the "relationships" as the feelings and interactions, both verbal and nonverbal, that occur among the members. In other words, a small group is conceived to be a system (Wells, 1990).

To be more specific, it is believed that a small group represents an *open system* (Barker, Wahlers, Watson, & Kibler, 1991) because it does not always maintain a steady state but is constantly developing and moving toward a steady state or homeostasis. This phenomenon of *homeostasis* is a useful concept to understand and to apply in the observation of the workings of a small group. It presupposes that the "individual," be it atom, cell, animal, or man, interacts with its environment and is governed by certain principles of equilibrium or homeostasis (Slavson, 1992). The individual has a preferred state of homeostasis and will consistently behave in a manner to maintain such a state. As the individual experiences the environment by behaving in certain ways, and experiences the behavior of others toward him, this state of equilibrium may be altered. Because of feelings of discomfort with this altered state and the need to return to the preferred state of equilibrium, the individual behaves in ways to try to bring this about (Rugel, 1991).

The same phenomenon occurs in a group. The group as an entity itself can be thought to desire a state of homeostasis. When any behavioral change occurs in a group member it affects every other member and hence the group as a whole (Barker, Wahlers, Watson, and Kibler, 1991). This precipitates reactionary behaviors in the other members in an attempt to regain a state of equilibrium or homeostasis (Slavson, 1992). Figure 2–1 is an example of how this process might be diagrammed.

Here, the group is depicted initially in a comfortable state and then when a group member says, "I'm feeling very sad," the other members immediately become activated to deal with the situation. They may try to explore why the member is feeling sad and they will almost surely offer advice on what could or should be done to overcome the sadness. A member is then most likely to be asked a question such as, "Has this discussion helped?" or "Are you feel-

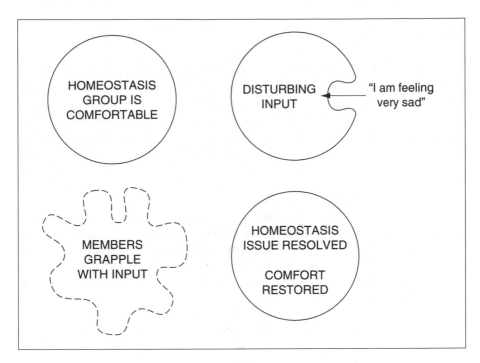

Figure 2–1. Maintenance of homeostasis among group members.

ing any better now?" This demonstrates the group's need to feel that the member is no longer sad and that they, including the distressed member, have returned to a state of equilibrium. One can usually tell when this state has been reached, as the group members appear to relax. You may even see an actual relaxing of body postures; members usually become quiet, even physically still, and seem to be in a rather tranquil state. Slavson (1992) refers to this state as "rest and recuperation."

This desire for a preferred state of comfort or balance can also be observed in the situation where the group appears to be comfortable but suddenly a member says something like, "I'm still upset by what John said to me." An interjection such as this will usually mobilize the group instantly. Members immediately query the member to determine what was said that was upsetting and then they are likely to query John to find out if he intended to be "upsetting." Through this process the members are really saying that they feel uncomfortable with this state of disequilibrium and they want to "fix" it so they can return to a more comfortable state. Not only may the presence of negative feelings cause members to react, but any intense situation, such as the sharing of intimate feelings or a deep emotional reaction, can elicit feelings of discomfort or embarrassment. Members then make efforts to regain a sense of balance in the emotional climate, as depicted in Figure 2–2, which is often attempted through an abrupt change of topic or focus.

The process just described encompasses the three perspectives from which Rapoport (1968) observes both living and nonliving systems. These fundamental aspects are structure, function, and evolution, or in terms more relative to a group's desire for equilibrium, being, action, and becoming. Looking again at Figure 2–2, the group can initially be seen to be in a state of "being." An "action" occurs, "I'm feeling very sad," which throws the group into the process of "becoming." No matter how the group functions at this stage it will eventually regain a state of being although this state will not be the same as before, because the group will have evolved to a new or different way of being (not necessarily better, only different).

In examining the world with all its complexities, it can be seen to be either one mammoth system or it can be seen as being made up of an infinite number of smaller systems. Hence some systems can be parts of a larger whole and can be called *subsystems* (Brown, 1993).

Now let us think in more practical and relevant terms. For example, consider an entity that most practitioners have had some experience with:

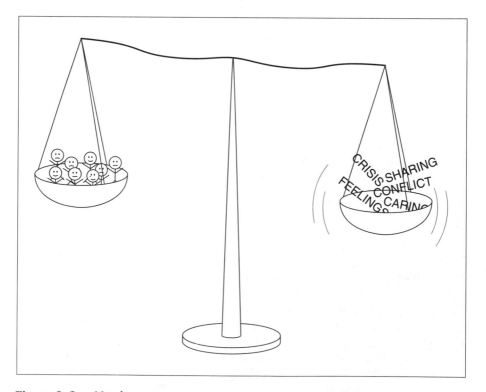

Figure 2–2. Members attempting to regain emotional balance.

a general hospital. The whole hospital may be regarded as a system, but it can also be thought of as comprising or encompassing many subsystems. Each department in the hospital can be seen as a system, as can each ward. Again, within each of these main entities there are likely to be many subsystems. Each ward has subsystems, such as the personnel on that ward or the overall treatment program. On examining the treatment program in Figure 2–3 we see that this subsystem also has subsystems—referred to here as sub-subsystems, one of which might be known as a small group or task group.

Other sub-subsystems of the treatment program might be the recreational program, the community program, or the chemotherapy treatment program. The small group may be a sub-subsystem of the overall treatment program subsystem, but it is also a system in and of itself with its own

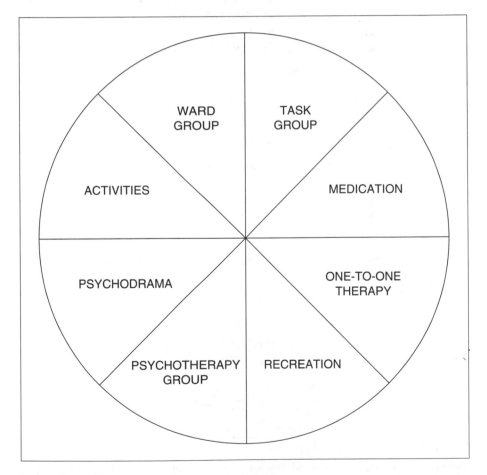

Figure 2–3.   Subsystems of treatment program.

subsystems. The subsystems of the small group are the individual members (Rugel, 1991).

Checkland (1981) presents a precise and detailed approach to defining systems by differentiating four classes as shown in Figure 2–4: (1) natural systems, (2) designed physical systems, (3) designed abstract systems, and (4) human activity systems. To see how the small group fits into this over-all classification a brief comment on each type of system is included here.

1. *Natural Systems.* These are physical systems that began at the origin of the universe. Their form was determined by the forces, processes, and evolution going on at that time, and their characteristics will remain the same as long as these determining factors remain the same. Thus the physical framework of the earth and other planets is considered to be a natural system. For example, the sun always rises in the east and sets in the

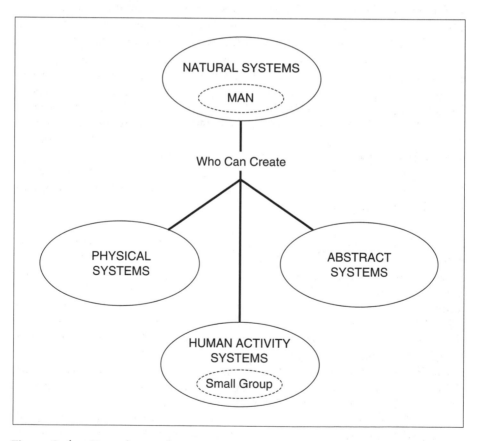

Figure 2–4.   Four classes of systems.

Source: Modified from P. Checkland. *Systems thinking, systems practice.* New York: Wiley, 1981.

west. The natural system of most relevance to our discussion is that of the human being: the person.

2. *Designed Physical Systems.* Such systems differ from natural systems in that they can be altered; they are the result of what humans have made by conscious design. They came about due to a need within or a perceived need, and so the point of their being is to serve a purpose. The telephone system designed by humans is a perfect example; it is one way to meet our desire for communication and, even at times, the need to survive. A concrete object like a book is also said to be a designed physical system; it has the purpose of preserving and disseminating information.

3. *Designed Abstract Systems.* If we look back to the previous example given to describe a designed physical system, that is, a book, it will lead us to an understanding of designed abstract systems. Being without physical properties, these systems evolve as conscious thoughts and ideas from humans' minds and are the stuff from which books, records, and films are made. Like the physical systems, they too serve a purpose, which might be the expansion of knowledge or the expression of the creative side of humans.

4. *Human Activity Systems.* This class of systems is the largest of the four and the one to which our entity of interest, a small group, belongs. Although these systems are not as tangible as the natural and designed systems, they are obvious entities with an underlying purpose. They consist of a number of activities related in a manner that gives the whole relevancy. In the case of the small group, the activities will be those of each group member as he relates to the productivity of the group and its goals. Although the small group is made up of human beings, which are themselves natural systems, the group as an entity is considered to be a human activity system: alternatively, a *system of systems*.

It is this concept of a whole and its parts that is of importance to those who lead or are involved in small groups. Douglas (1991) points out that one must be aware of this system of systems because the group cannot be completely isolated from its environment and can be affected by the larger system, of which it forms a part, in any number of ways. Leaders must also be aware that their group is made up of several members, each of whom has his or her own individuality, expressed or not expressed as needs, wishes, fears, or caring. Although these members or subsystems, when together, do form a whole or system (i.e., the group), it is very important to constantly be aware of and sensitive to their functioning as individuals. It can be difficult for a leader to do this consistently.

Take, for example, a decision-making group where the goal or task for a given session is to rank order a list of attributes by the process of consensus. As the group begins, there is a lively discussion by most members, and it can be easy for the leader to get caught up in the content or productivity of the large system while ignoring one or more of the subsystems (individual members). It may appear as if the group or large system is functioning well as it moves quickly and perhaps efficiently toward the completion of the task. On close observation of the individuals, however, it might be the case that one member is not participating at all.

It can be easy to miss such an occurrence if the leader is focusing almost exclusively on the larger system. She needs to be aware of all the subsystems, sensitive to their individuality and to their unique needs and ways of functioning and expressing themselves. Because each individual has input into the group (even lack of input is input), the total system will be affected. These initial and ongoing actions and interactions meld into a process that can be observed and compartmentalized as the group develops.

THE PROCESS OF GROUP DEVELOPMENT

Similar to the way Eric Erikson (1963) set out his theory of the stages of development in a person, theorists have described developmental stages for groups. We refer to a group as having a life of its own and just as each human life is different from others so is each group, and each session of any specified group, different from others. A group is not a static thing but rather it ebbs and flows in different ways and at different paces. Just as a person's development can be arrested at a certain stage, so too can a group plateau for a time at a certain stage or regress to an earlier stage. The question is whether there is any consistent form to the changes that occur in groups. Are there definitive stages that a group passes through on its way to becoming a functioning unit, and do all groups move through the same stages? Unfortunately there are no easy answers to these questions since the paucity of new research on group development leaves the work of the seventies or earlier as the main source and basis for discussion (Gersick, 1988). It is not clear if this lack is an endorsement of the early work or a lack of research interest in this topic area.

McCollom (1990) calls into question the validity of several of the early models on the basis that they have generalized group development across all types of groups. In addition she points out weaknesses and discrepancies in the types of data collected and the methods of analysis used to evaluate disparate types of groups in order to generalize to a "model fits all" position. She notes that task and problem-solving groups differ significantly from therapy or T-groups but that these differences were ignored in an effort to present a generalized group development model. It is believed, however, that Tuckman's (1965) life-cycle model, which seems to have survived the test of time, to some degree addresses these differences by examining group processes as they relate to structure, task, and therapeutic aspects. The important concept for group leaders to grasp is that groups are constantly changing and that there appears to be similar and recognizable stages of development that occur in all groups. The answer is that all groups do experience different stages although the boundaries are vague at times and groups may function in overlapping stages.

The Authority Cycle

This perspective presents the stages of group development in terms of the relationship between the leader and group members. It describes the feelings, behavior, and movement of group members as being directly related to the behavior of the leader. At the beginning of the cycle or development of the group, authority is seen as being vested in the leader. As the group develops, this authority is gradually transferred from the leader to the members. This is not always a smooth passage, and as can be seen in Figure 2–5, there are several stages.

Dependence The first stage of the authority cycle is that of *dependence* (A). This is the starting point of most groups and at this point the members are dependent on the leader for direction and total support. There is little if any interaction between members as they look to the leader to tell them what to do and explain what is expected of them. Gemmill (1986) uses the term *deskill* to describe how group members embrace what he refers to as the "leader-myth," by denying their own abilities and resources to perform and function independently as a group. He portrays the members as projecting

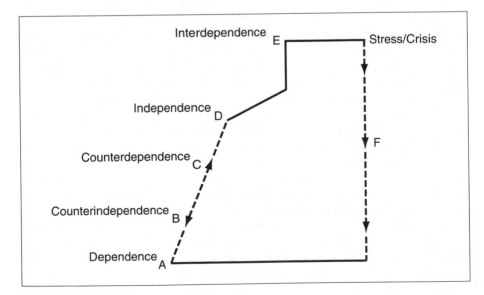

Figure 2–5. Stages of the authority cycle.

all their coping and creative skills onto the designated leader. By deskilling themselves the members strengthen the authority of the leader and reinforce their own feelings of confusion, helplessness, and dependency. As the leader tries to move out of this authoritative role by offering the group its free-dom—freedom of choice, freedom to decide, freedom to make the group their own, the group's initial reaction is often one of hostility.

Counterindependence   Members prefer a comfortable structural situa-tion where they are told what to do over one where they experience the in-security of having to accept responsibility. This stage is known as the *coun-terindependence* stage (B) and the general feeling in the group is one of fear and anger. Members are hostile to the leader because she is not living up to their expectations (Sklare, Keener, & Mas, 1990). The leader is not telling them what to do, organizing, or doing things for them. Generally, in their eyes she is not being a "good leader." Srivastva and Barrett (1988) metaphor-ically refer to this stage of a group as a "rudderless ship."

Counterdependence   When the group finally accepts the fact that it has some freedom to make decisions and determine its own life, it begins to move away from the leader; this stage is known as *counterdependence* (C). This stage is often characterized by a struggle for authority and leadership among the members (Verdi & Wheelan, 1992). As the members realize that the established leader is not going to do the job, group members begin to assert themselves by vying for the role. This movement away from the leader is often accompanied by expressions of hostility ("All right, if you aren't going to do the job we'll show you"), or rejection ("We can get along without you"). At this point the group tries to establish some norms and patterns of operation which will provide the stability they need to function independently of the leader. If the leader does not grant the group free-dom to express its hostility, the group may stifle its anger, become resis-tive, and group growth may be inhibited. The leader must be willing to suf-fer the discomfort of some rejection and hostility in order to help the group progress to accepting responsibility for itself. This stage is usually one of tension and strain. The group therefore is not very creative and morale may be low.

Independence   If the leader accepts the group's declaration of indepen-dence displayed in the counterdependence stage, then the group is free to enter a new phase of its existence which is known as the stage of *indepen-dence* (D). This stage is usually a joyful one for the group. As they experience their freedom and independence they may take flight from reality through laughter and giddiness. The leader may experience a feeling of being left out as the general attitude of the members is one of ignoring the leader. Mem-bers frequently behave in ways that convey, "See, we don't need you; we can do this by ourselves." Frequently at this stage, members resist getting on with the business of the group, as they enjoy their independence, the heightened morale of the group, and their new feelings of togetherness. The group begins to feel strong as a unit, and as a result of this, members display increased confidence and comfort.

Interdependence As these feelings of confidence and unity among the members strengthen, the members stop fighting the leader and permit her to reenter the group. This is done by listening to and accepting any contributions now made by the leader. Because the group experiences a sense of control over what is happening, this feeling is extended to allow the leader to participate. This sense of control that members feel also allows them to feel safe in their relationships with one another and paves the way for the group to move on to the *interdependence* stage (E). At this stage members interact in equal, encouraging, and supportive ways with one another and with the leader.

As Stockton, Rohde, and Haughey (1992) note, however, groups tend to "shift from earlier to later stages and then back again" (p. 164). This back-and-forth movement, although it may occurr within a group's overall linear development, has been referred to as the *pendular* or *recurring cycle* model of development (Berman-Rossi, 1992). As long as there are no undue events or pressures on the group, it may continue to function productively and creatively at the stage of interdependence. However, should a crisis or something untoward occur (even something as benign as a new member joining the group), then the group may fall back (F) to the stage of dependence (A) with a "How do we handle this?" or "What do we do now?" approach to the leader.

The leader's response to such an occurrence is crucial to the continued functional health of the group. A leader may intentionally or unintentionally welcome the dependence and move to actively take over the group again by telling them to "do this" or "do that." If the leader follows this with further directive behavior, she will find the group entrenched again at the dependence stage, in effect back at square one. However, the leader who responds to the crisis event at the interdependent stage with a problem-solving approach enables the group to maintain its interdependent functional abilities. Rather than telling the members what they should do, the leader might ask, "What do you think we should do?," "What alternatives do we have?," "What might help?" By engaging in this problem-solving approach with the members the leader is emphasizing the interdependence of members with one another and with the leader. The leader is also giving the members a message of faith in their functional abilities: a message that says "I'll help, but I also need your help and together we can work this out."

If a group does revert back to an earlier stage of development, it is often for a brief period of time. Each time this happens the group is likely to move more rapidly through the ensuing stages or they may even jump directly back to interdependence without experiencing the intervening stages.

The time it takes for any given group to progress through the stages varies greatly (Hare, 1992). Some groups will go through the process very rapidly in the first session, others less rapidly over a couple of sessions, and still other groups may evolve gradually over several sessions. The process depends on many variables such as (a) leadership style and skill; (b) the characteristics of the members, including personality and ability; (c) environmental circumstances; (d) the purpose of the group; and (e) the duration and number of sessions of the group. Now let us examine these variables more closely.

VARIABLES AFFECTING GROUP DEVELOPMENT

Leadership Style and Skill

It is obvious that a leader's style and skill will affect the development of any group. A leader who likes to make all the decisions as to what the group is to do and when, and who likes to keep close control of the group, will find that the group is likely to remain in the dependent stage. Because all groups start at this stage and members may have no other experience, they are apt to be compliant and continue to do what they are told without question. As will be noted later in the discussion of leadership styles, members under authoritarian leadership rarely have the opportunity to make decisions nor are they usually given any responsibility. For some members, such as those who are depressed, such a situation is quite acceptable. But it can be seen that such an environment is not conducive to individuals becoming motivated, energized, or empowered to take responsibility for their lives and behaviors.

A democratic leader, on the other hand, usually encourages the members to become actively involved and stresses the attainment of an interdependent environment among group members and between group members and herself. In this role the leader tries to move out of the position of control and willingly accepts members' behaviors that are inherent in the stages of counterinterdependence, counterdependence, and independence, in order for the group to evolve to a state of interdependence. This is done by being patient, accepting, responsive, tolerant, and good-natured, and by being aware of one's feelings and dealing with them within oneself. For example, when the group is floundering and the leader experiences great frustration, she controls the urge to jump in and say "Do this" or "Do it that way." Rather the leader lets the group struggle until they figure it out "their way." This is not to say that the leader cannot offer information or encouragement or be supportive, but only to say that she does not do it for them. To do this requires many of the skills discussed under leadership skills.

Characteristics of the Members

Often the progression of a group through its stages of development depends mainly on the functional level of the members (MacKenzie & Livesley, 1983). If a group is made up primarily of depressed individuals, it will be extremely difficult to facilitate movement past the dependent stage. Rarely will they have the energy to be actively hostile, as is characteristic of the counterdependence stage, so when offered choices they are likely to respond with apathy or complete withdrawal. These are less obvious forms of hostility but ones that ensure a state of dependence. In such a situation the leader is forced to again become motivator, activator, and decision maker.

Conversely, if the membership includes many overconfident, verbal members, they may be more than willing to accept or even seize control of the group from the leader. However, they may then become bogged down with infighting and one-upmanship in attempts to secure a single leadership position. This can prevent the group from moving on to interdependence and more group-shared productivity.

As a leader it is important to be aware of the characteristics of members and to adjust one's expectations and behavior accordingly. Also, a group does not have to be in the interdependent stage to be a useful group. To have very depressed members respond to directions and participate, even if minimally and in a dependent way, may be an enormous progression for them. Groups, with chronic, low-functioning members, may remain at this basic level but can continue to be useful in the important and therapeutic role of maintenance. Usually leaders find they have a mix of functional levels among members which in and of itself can monitor and have facilitative effects.

Environment

As is discussed later in the book, the environment plays a crucial role in the progress of any group. Many groups, especially therapy groups, meet in hospitals where the medical model prevails. This model embodies the idea of being "done to." Patients are given medicines, food, housing, and rules, and in general are "looked after." They have little say about any of the aspects of their stay, so it is not surprising that when they come to a group they resist (counterindependence) having to take responsibility to make decisions. Many want to be "cured" and they expect the leader to do this, just as they have invested the physician with the ability and the responsibility to do this. In such an environment it takes skill and perseverance to work at inducing responsibility and motivating independent behaviors.

Purpose of the Group

The purpose or goals of a life-skills group, for example, will differ in character from those of a classical psychotherapy group. In a life-skills group, because the purpose will be to help the members learn or relearn some discreet behaviors, the leader is likely to maintain somewhat of a teacher–leader role. Because the leader has information to be imparted to the members, be it scenarios to be role-played or instructions on specific activities or techniques, this inequality of functions (teacher–learner) will keep the members in somewhat dependent roles vis-à-vis the leader for a longer period of time. In the psychotherapy group, where the goals are more vague and abstract, the leader may be completely nondirective right from the beginning. This can create high levels of anxiety in the members, putting them immediately into the counterindependence stage. A third example, that of a decision making or consensus group, may help to clarify the point. The leader may give the group a list of variables to be rank ordered according to certain principles. The group may quickly embrace the task and begin making decisions by majority vote. The leader may try to intervene to get the group to make decisions through discussion, but the suggestion is rejected because the group has quickly moved to the counterdependence stage, and although they may be vying for leadership among themselves, they are united in wanting to do it their way.

Duration and Number of Sessions

Each consecutive group session involving the same individuals is likely to present more independent and interdependent behaviors among the members than did the previous session. It is usual for cohesion and trust to increase from one session to the next, forming an emotional climate conducive to assuming responsibility and working together. This progression encourages members to move forward through the various stages thus facilitating group development.

The duration of any one session will affect the degree to which members become familiar and trusting of one another and consequently their willingness to take risks and to function in independent ways. Sessions of less than one hour do not allow sufficient time for warm-up or closure (Gladding, 1991) or for any degree of trust to develop, and they tend to encourage members to rely on the leader for direction.

It can be seen from these examples that there are many variables which can affect the nature and pace of the development of a group. Because of these variables the rate of passage varies widely with different groups and even within each session of the same group.

STAGES OF DEVELOPMENT

There are several models delineating group development (Berman-Rossi, 1992) and all suggest a "progressive" movement of the group as a whole.

Much of the literature in this area recognizes the work of Tuckman (1965) as presenting one of the first models to conceptualize the sequential behavior changes that occur throughout the life cycle of a small group. His model includes four phases: *inclusion, control, affection,* and *functional—* also referred to as *forming, storming, norming,* and *performing.* In a later work, Tuckman and Jensen (1977) suggest that a fifth phase, *adjournment,* be added to the model. This stage of a group, also called the termination stage by others (Braaten, 1974/1975; Keyton, 1993), is addressed in Chapter 11.

Lacoursiere (1980) refers to the stages of development as *orientation, dissatisfaction, resolution, production,* and *termination*—names which are fairly descriptive of the behaviors, thoughts, and feelings that are occurring in the group at each of the stages. Lacoursiere brings our attention to the fact that a developmental sequence is present in all types of groups although this has mostly been discussed in the context of therapy groups. He notes that organizational groups, learning groups, treatment teams, sometimes classrooms, and even "falling in love" all display developmental stages.

As a leader, the usefulness of being aware of the developmental process of a group is to help understand the dynamics in the group at any given time. This is especially comforting at times when the group appears to be floundering or upset and these feelings and behaviors can be related to a specific developmental stage. This is not to say that leaders can relax and depend on the stages to take care of the group's progress. A sensitive and aware leader can facilitate the group's coping with some of the stresses inherent in a group's development and monitor the members' passage through the ups and downs of a group's life.

Orientation Stage

According to Schultz (1986), the main concerns of members in the initial phase of any group are personally centered and have to do with the issue of belonging. Members' feelings reflect such concerns as, "Will I be accepted?" . . . "Will the others like me?" . . . "Do I know as much as the others?" . . . "If I speak will anyone listen?" . . . "Will I be different?" . . . "What will the leader think of me?" Members deal with these anxious feelings by testing or trying out different behaviors in order to size up the situation. Seashore (1974) sees this stage as one where members form "collusive relationships" in an effort to establish some form of security. Members may be overtalkative or withdrawn, display a self-centered unawareness and insensitivity to others, try to impress the group by talking about outside experiences, display attention-getting behaviors, and pressure others into taking responsibility. Ferencik (1992) notes that members may be passive during this initial stage due to "structural ambiguity"—that is, members do not clearly understand the respective roles of leaders and members.

If a task has been suggested, group members initially avoid taking responsibility for any decision making concerning the task. Member input abounds with such comments or questions as "I don't know," "What do the rest of you think?," "How long do we have to do it?," "Are we to work together?" Someone might then suggest, "Well, let's go around the table and everyone can give a suggestion." The next suggestion or question might be, "Shall we vote on the different ideas?"

Through all this the group is trying to discover how they are going to approach the task, what they need to know, and how decisions are going to be made. Frequently questions will be directed to the leader, for guidance (dependence) and as a means of checking out the ground rules.

In therapy groups Tuckman (1965) reports behaviors characterizing this stage as being, in part, (a) griping about the institutional environment, (b) discussing peripheral problems, (c) discussing symptoms, (d) searching for the meaning of therapy, (e) attempting to establish rapport with the therapist, (f) intellectualizing, and (g) being suspicious and fearful of the new situation. In essence, the members of a therapy group at this stage are attempting to determine what will be expected of them, what they can expect to gain, whom they can relate to, and who is going to help them. For these reasons clients need plenty of time to go through these initial explorations, and it is a mistake to hurry them or force them into close contact with others before they are ready (Battegay, 1986).

Dissatisfaction Stage

The outstanding characteristics of this stage are frustration, conflict, lack of unity, and testing-out behaviors. Even if the orientation stage has been handled well, the social-emotional aspects of this stage can be disruptive and difficult (Lacoursiere, 1980). If the leader abdicates the leadership role in favor of the group assuming responsibility, then hostile feelings will develop between members and the leader. Members feel lost and uncertain ("Are we doing this the right way?" . . . "What is the right way?" . . . "Who is going to make the decisions?" . . . "Who is going to tell us what to do?"). In order to deal with such anxieties some members will try to make the decisions ("I think we should do . . . " "What we should do now is . . . " "Let's just pick a topic and get started"). At this point the interaction in the group may become uneven as some members withdraw, especially if they have made a suggestion and no one picked up on it; other members may disagree with such suggestions as they are put forth and offer or not offer their own, while still others will compete for the leadership position seen to be abandoned by the leader. One observes competition rather than cooperation. Each member is trying to express individuality but often shys away from decision making or from accepting responsibility for the group's actions.

Members display an emotional response to any task and their reactions are frequently negative ("Who wants to do this anyway?" . . . "This is kid's stuff" . . . "We did this in kindergarten" . . . "This is dumb"). Bion, (1961) describes this period in a group as one of *fight–flight*. Most often he used the term to describe the interactions between the group and the leader, where members entered into conflict with the leader or they tried to withdraw psychologically from the whole situation. However, the term can also be applied to interactions among the group members when conflict or discord is present.

During this stage in therapy groups members tend to become argumentative, anxious, ambivalent toward the leader, and negative toward the group (Tuckman, 1965). Some acting out may occur as members are not sure of one another and are wary of the leader. Because of their fears and anxieties, at this point, members are more concerned with what seems to them to be self-preservation than they are with treatment.

Fortunately for all involved, group development is such that invariably members not only survive the struggles of this phase, but gradually the very process they are involved in moves the group on to the next phase. As the group struggles in this stage, it may be helpful for the leader to initiate a discussion of the goals of the group and to present the developmental stages to the members to help them understand the process that is occurring.

Resolution Stage

This stage may not be as definitive as the previous stage but may "start with a decrease in dissatisfaction at one end, and extend to neutral or clearly positive feelings at the other end" (Lacoursiere, 1980, p. 32). It is characterized by members beginning to listen to what others are saying resulting in the gradual development of consensual validation, group unity, and cohesion. However, there can be some negative feelings toward a member (or members) who is not responsive to the positive overtures being expressed. With harmony being a goal at this point, members have low tolerance for those who do not support this norm. Members generally feel good about themselves and about the group. Positive feelings and comments are prevalent ("I like your idea . . . " "You are good at . . . " "I am . . . " "How shall we do . . . ?" "How do you feel about . . . ?" "Let's . . . ").

Trust increases leading to genuine openness and sharing. As some members begin to disclose and confide personal information, others feel more comfortable in revealing themselves. Questioning and probing becomes an accepted norm. Members feel safe.

Production Stage

By the time it reaches this phase, the group has developed to a point where trust is high and members feel free to get on with the group in a unified manner (Schroder & Harvey, 1963) without the emotional interference of anxieties. Various members may assume directive roles at different times and these leadership functions are welcomed although not necessarily always acted on. The atmosphere in the group is a productive one, one of give and take.

In a task group, with the problem-solving techniques that have emerged and using the information shared and evaluated in the previous phases, solutions emerge as to how the task will be accomplished. At this stage the group can become caught up in the task and seem to have a vested interest in its completion. The members are now working collaboratively as a unit in an interdependent manner toward achieving the task and this goal becomes their main focus.

Termination

This final stage of the group is a time of consolidation. It is during this time that members review their experience, achieve understanding and insight, and analyze some of their problems. Members must also "dissolve their ties" with one another as they prepare for a state of "grouplessness" (Berman-Rossi, 1993). This is also a time of looking to the future and this stage emphasizes the transfer of learning from the group to real life (Matthews, 1992). In task groups this last stage also often constitutes a discussion of how the task evolved, feedback to one another, how different members felt and what roles they played during the task, and what members learned about themselves and how they might do things differently. The format used in these groups will depend on the type of task that is introduced.

One format is for the members to work on a shared activity by themselves without any input from or intervention by the leader. She will usually remain in the group or sit close by in order to observe the process and to intervene should it be necessary. Then when the group indicates they have finished or if their time is up, the leader initiates a discussion. The discussion, as mentioned earlier, should involve an evaluation of how the group functioned during the activity. Depending on the nature of the activity the discussion may touch on issues such as division of tasks and responsibilities, how members felt at different points during the activity, how members reacted to and interacted with one another, and what could have been done differently.

Another format is for the leader to take an active role in the group throughout. In this case the leader comments on the process and intervenes as the group progresses. The leader makes observations, points out behaviors, encourages members to participate and share their feelings, gives feedback, and generally tries to get the members to examine the *when, what, where,* and *how* of the happenings during the session. A third format is for each member to do the task individually, such as a drawing or collage, and then when finished to share what they have done with the rest of the group. In this case it is usually best if the leader does the activity with the members.

This gives her the opportunity to be aware of what the members are experiencing, be a role model for performing the task, downplay the leadership role, and be able to observe what is going on in the group without appearing to be sitting and watching.

Not every group will move through the stages as clearly and smoothly as has been presented here but rather, as with human development, each group will do so at its own speed. As noted in the discussion of the authority cycle, groups can also get bogged down at any one stage or revert back to an earlier stage. It should be noted that the type of task the group is involved in is not usually an issue in group development. Different tasks may bring about different dynamics (e.g., taking turns, working individually at times) but the developmental sequence will basically follow the same pattern. Only the rate of development and the time spent in the various stages may differ.

SUMMARY

A small group meets the requirements of a system by having members as the "parts," the personalities of the members as the "properties," and the feelings and interactions among the members as the "relationships." In addition, a group is believed to be an open system because it does not maintain a constant state of homeostasis but is constantly developing and changing. In considering the four types of systems—natural, designed physical, designed abstract, and human activity—small groups fall into the last category.

Any ongoing group is in a constant process of development. The rate and nature of this development depends on several variables such as the skill and style of leadership, the characteristics of the members, the environment, the purpose of the group, the length of the group, the interactions among the members, and the interactions between the leader and the members. These variables will be of more or less importance in the development of different groups.

Group development encompasses distinct stages. The model presented here includes five stages—orientation, dissatisfaction, resolution, production, and termination. At each of these stages it can be informative and useful to direct observations along three parameters. By focusing on the three parameters—group structure, task behaviors, and therapy—an observer is more likely to be aware of all aspects of the group's development. Although most groups grapple with all five stages, each group does so in different ways and within a different time frame.

Chapter 3

Group Dimensions

*All groups require warmth and
protection—some more than others.*
— ALFRED BENJAMIN

Quite different from the structured and formalized phase development approach to group development is Dimock's (1985a) framework of group dimensions. He emphasizes the importance of understanding the factors that affect the development or growth of a group as a means of guiding one's observations of process. Dimock states that "by observing, understanding and giving attention to these areas groups can improve their procedures, accomplish higher level tasks, and enable members to satisfy more of their developmental needs" (Dimock, 1985a, p. 1). For Dimock this framework takes the form of five dimensions: *climate, interaction, involvement, cohesion,* and *productivity*. This chapter discusses all five areas. The climate or environment of a group is a first consideration, and because it is the one component that can be directly affected by the attentiveness of the leader, this component is given special emphasis.

CLIMATE

Most people concern themselves with the state of the living room, family room, or recreation room whenever they are going to have friends over. It is usual to want the room to appear inviting, look tidy and attractive, and, hopefully, be comfortable. For the same reasons, group leaders should be equally concerned with the group room before members arrive. Barris (1982) concludes that the environment can play a role in affecting a person in three areas: developing interests and values, communicating performance expectations, and affecting participation in future environments. The surroundings in which a group is held can exert the same effects and can have a strong influence on the group process (Gladding, 1991; Palazzolo, 1981).

Unfortunately, this is an aspect that is often ignored or overlooked by leaders. Some leaders are not aware of the importance of the environment to the overall functioning of the group. Others were aware at one time but through habit, work constraints, familiarity, or carelessness, they have ceased to see this as an area of focus or concern. Still others have a sense that "things have always worked this way so why change?" The leader needs to be sensitive at all times to dynamics in the group that may be a result of environmental factors. Such factors can have an effect at any time so the leader should keep this possibility in mind throughout the group, not only at the beginning.

Environmental Factors

There are two major environmental factors to consider: (1) physical factors and (2) emotional factors (Dimock, 1985a). Under physical factors the following are discussed here: (a) space, (b) temperature, (c) seating arrangements, (d) sound, and (e) dress. Emotional factors involve the mood of (a) the leader, (b) the group, and (c) individual members of the group.

Physical Factors

Space The amount of space available and how it is utilized is of utmost importance in setting up a group. Levine (1979) suggests "the room where the group meets and its set-up can greatly enhance or distract from the group's development" (p. 7). Ideally, you will be in a position to select and furnish the room in which you will hold your group. Realistically, you will probably be allotted the room or the space. Most likely, you will hold your group in a room that is used by different staff members at various times for other activities such as meetings, individual sessions, other groups, and social events.

Given the ideal situation, what kind of selections should you make? Some group leaders feel that if you have windows in your room you will have noise and distractions. This may be true for certain situations, but it is the writer's belief that the light and feeling of openness more than compensates for these drawbacks. If you have a bright, windowed room, you are more likely to induce a "bright" group. A windowless room tends to give a dingy, closed-in feeling, which in turn is apt to encourage only a "closed" unproductive group.

Space is an important factor to consider when setting up your group (Nelson-Jones, 1992; Saint-Jean & Desrosiers, 1993). You will need enough space so that you can organize your group comfortably either around a table or seated in a circle without a table. A sectioned table is sometimes useful— when it is not needed, it can be easily set aside in the unused corners of the room rather than take up most of one end or side of the room. You also will need enough space for group members to space themselves comfortably apart from one another and not feel their personal space is invaded. However, you do want members seated close enough together so that interaction is encouraged. You also need to keep in mind that you may want to easily manoeuvre extra chairs in and out of the group, say, for role-playing.

Like Goldilocks, for the *ideal* situation, you want a room that is not too big and not too small. Too large a room can detract from feelings of closeness and cohesion and too small a room can cause members to feel hemmed in or trapped (Corey, Corey, Callanan, & Russell, 1992). Often, leaders solve the problem of a large space by organizing one corner of the room into the group area. In doing so the leader provides walls and hence "protection" on at least two sides of the group and thus a little more sense of security for the members.

Space problems can also be related to scheduling and the needs of other staff members. The situation can arise where the room in which you routinely hold your sessions has been appropriated by another staff member for a special presentation. On discovering this conflict in scheduling it may be suggested that you could hold your group in the "small room across from the office." The problem this presents is one of *territoriality*, not in the sense of your territory as a professional (although this could be an issue) but in the sense of the group members' territory. When hospitalized, clients give up the familiar territory of their homes and all their personal places such as "my room," "my place at the table," "my closet," and so on. In a hospital they establish new territories, spaces, and places which they can feel are theirs. The group room can have meaning in this context as a place they are familiar with and feel comfortable in. Addressing this point, Battegay (1986) says the room does not merely belong to the group; it is a part of it (p. 143). He goes on to emphasize the importance of establishing a group room that remains constant. So before accepting the quick solution of the room across from the office, it would be in the best interests of the group to pursue the issue for alternatives that offer a better choice. Some options might be:

- Try to get the group that is having the presentation in the group room to relocate.
- Try to find a room that is similar to the regular group room. Perhaps the room across from the office is not the only room to consider.
- Hold the group at a different time but in the usual room.

Holding the group in the small available room is probably a better alternative than another possible option which is to cancel the group for that day. Should you decide to cancel the session, be sure you or a reliable staff member contact each member to inform them of the circumstances and the reasons for the cancellation. Some members will be disappointed and others may feel relieved. Either way they need a full explanation, preferably from the group leader or another staff member. If it can be avoided, do not ask a group member to tell the other members; this can raise all sorts of brooding questions in the minds of the members. They also may feel that the group cannot be very important if you do not take the time to inform them of the change yourself.

Temperature   It goes without saying that the room needs to be well ventilated with a comfortable temperature. The latter may be quite difficult to achieve for all group members. Some members may prefer a cooler room than others due to their medication or their natural preference. It is quite usual for older clients to prefer a warm room temperature. It is a good idea to check this out with your members and not rely totally on your own comfort level or preference. A room that is very warm is likely to cause clients to feel groggy and not too energetic or motivated.

If you are conducting a group session that will require physical movement, such as an exercise group or even an active warm-up exercise, it is important to be aware of the temperature factor and try to adjust it to the needs of the group. Opening a window or the door while engaged in these sorts of activities usually does not cause any disruption to the group.

Seating Arrangements   How and where clients sit in a group may appear to be very mundane issues. In actual fact, they are issues of consequence and can greatly affect the dynamics in the group (Brandler & Roman, 1991). The type of seats, how they are arranged, and where clients choose to sit are all significant issues and require the attention of the group leader. Research by Pellegrini (1971) demonstrates that sitting at the head of a rectangular table can have a significant effect on all the other persons seated at the table. He found that the person who occupies the end position was rated higher on dimensions such as talkativeness, dominance, persuasiveness, self-confidence, leadership, and intelligence. Looking at Figure 3–1 one can see how all the group members are focused on the man seated at the end of the table.

It is also interesting to note how the members seated distant from the focal person tend to lean forward in attempts to be included. As leader of a small group where you wish to encourage participation and downplay your authority role, it is particularly important to avoid sitting in this head position yourself. Unfortunately, members will invariably avoid this seat too, leaving it for the leader. In this case it is best to ask a member to switch places with you before starting the group.

Type of Seats   Most members coming into a group look for the most comfortable chair. For the majority of group members, this translates into the softest chair! So, if you have a variety of seats for members to sit on, such as easy chairs, sofas, armchairs, straight-backed chairs, and stools, you will probably find that the first members to arrive will head for the relaxation of the easy chairs and sofa. A relaxed setting can also encourage "relaxed" behavior which is not always positive. This was demonstrated when co-leaders of a life-skills group with young offenders agreed to have their third session

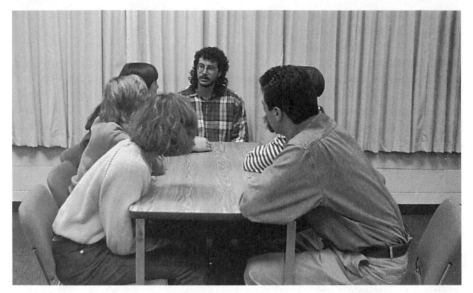

Figure 3–1.   Focus of members when one of the group sits in the head position.

in the facility's lounge. This room, furnished with sofas and easy chairs, was very familiar to the young offenders as this was where they spent much of their leisure time. In their post-group analysis of the session, the leaders could not decide if it was the seating in the room or the usual use factor (e.g., lounging) that precipitated an unproductive session that was disrupted by noise, horseplay, inattention, conflict, and other excitable behaviors. They concluded it was a combination of both factors. For the next session they returned to the room used previously and sat in a circle on hard-backed chairs; the leaders were relieved to experience a cooperative, interactive, more focused group.

Levels   As can be observed in Figure 3–2, when you have a mixture of chairs and sofas of different types, the actual seating surfaces vary in heights; hence, your members will be sitting at different levels. This "up-and-down" situation affects the interactions in the group (Nelson-Jones, 1992) as well as how members feel toward one another. Take the situation where a member is feeling depressed or particularly down and is seated in a soft, low-cushioned easy chair or even on the floor, beside a member on a solid straight-backed and thus a higher-level chair. The discrepancy in the levels of the two members tends to accentuate the situation and may cause the lower-level member to feel even more depressed or down. The best one can do is to have all the chairs the group uses be similar, if not the same type. This removes competition for the soft seats, any distractions caused by "who is sitting in which chair," and problems related to differences in eye levels.

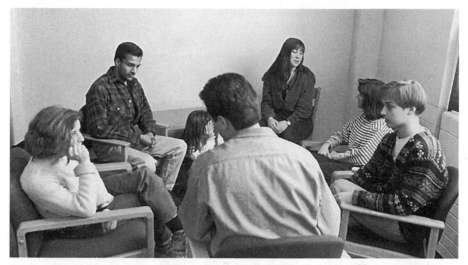

Figure 3–2.   "Unevenness" of members caused by different sitting heights.

Sitting on pillows on the floor, as shown in Figure 3–3, may lesson the formality of the group and promote intimacy. However, even a difference in pillows can be an issue as happened in a group led by the author and a co-therapist. Because the experience was to be a weekend group, the plan was to sit on pillows on the floor in the hopes of being more comfortable. Twelve large pillows covered in material of a blue-and-black design were available and just the right number for the expected twelve group members. The co-leaders, realizing the need for two more pillows, picked up two available sleeping pillows and took them along to sit on, and they began the group. Being bed pillows, both had ordinary white pillowcases. The group was slower getting started than had been expected; the members seemed a little tense and tentative. After about an hour, a member finally asked what was the meaning behind the white pillows the leaders were sitting on. As soon as the question was asked, the group came alive with many other members joining in the querying. It was obvious that most group members had been concerned and preoccupied with the pillows from the beginning of the session. Once it was explained that the white pillows held no significance the tone of the group became more relaxed and comfortable.

Configuration   Make every effort to have your group members seated in a circle (Figure 3–4), as this encourages and facilitates communication among the members. Figuratively speaking, a circle is a symbol of inclusion and closeness (Grady, 1994). Heap (1977) notes that "interaction is most likely to occur where participants are able to see each other" (p. 122). Verbal

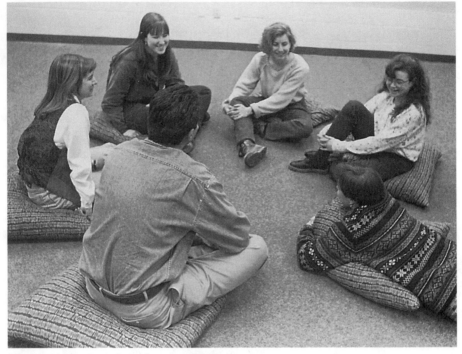

Figure 3–3.   An informal atmosphere.

groups are most always seated in a circle without a table. However, task groups, where members are involved in doing an activity, tend to be conducted with members seated around a table, as shown in Figure 3–5. In this situation the table is mainly utilitarian, supplying a surface for members to work on while carrying out the task's requirements.

In discussing the pros and cons of using tables in groups, Levine (1979) notes that a table can have several other useful purposes. It offers support to group members, it gives them something to lean on, a place to put their hands, and serves as a link between the group members. In groups with children or adolescents a table can often serve as a divider to keep antagonistic members separated and thereby reduce opportunities for physical contact. Finally, members who are feeling shy, self-conscious, or nervous may find the table to be partial protection from physically exposing themselves to others. If it is decided that a table should be used, then the importance of finding a round table must be emphasized even though it seems that the tables available in most facilities tend to be rectangular.

By looking at Figure 3–6 on page 43, one can see how the seating configuration can affect the type of interactions that occur. With this rectangular positioning and eight members, one can see that two subgroups—A-B-C

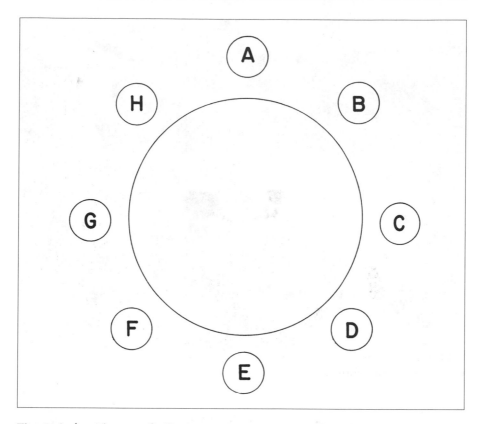

Figure 3–4. The most facilitative seating arrangement for group members.

and F-G-H—may be formed. This possibility exists because members will most often talk to (a) someone they can easily make eye contact with, or (b) someone who is sitting close to them (Finlay, 1993). These two tenets hold true for the three members of each of the two subgroups. This does not mean the subgroups will be active at the same time during the session, but when members in these locations do interact, it is likely to be in the directions indicated. It may be argued that G is also close to E or that D is close to B. This is true, of course, but the second tenet does not hold true for these pairs because they cannot make eye contact easily. In Figure 3–7 on page 44, the two members in the center on the sofas appear left out of the conversation and are too distant from each other to interact comfortably. To make eye contact is really what we mean when we say "I can see you," and if we say "I can't see you," we usually mean, "I can't see your eyes."

It is true that some people have difficulty making or maintaining eye contact, but even persons who do find it difficult to make eye contact like to know the other person involved is facing them so that if they do glance up

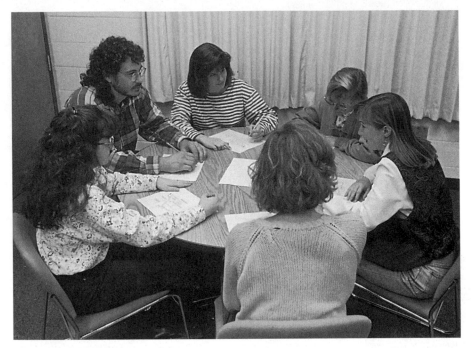

Figure 3–5.   Doing an activity.

they feel some contact. There is more opportunity and it is much easier for members to make eye contact when seated in a circle. It can be seen in Figure 3–8 on page 45 that the angles between each group member from, for example, the position of E, are almost equal. These angles would be the same for the other members in relation to the rest of the group as well.

Sound   Often a group leader is at the mercy of the physical layout of the department or facility in terms of finding a suitable room in which to hold group sessions. Rarely does a department enjoy the luxury of having a special group room. Surrounding sounds that may not disrupt the other activities a room is used for are often very distracting if one is conducting a group. Sometimes a group room is formed by separating a large room with a divider of some sort such as a folding wall. Although such dividers may remove visual distractions, they do not keep out the sound of music, voices, or laughter. Noise can be disruptive as well as make it difficult for members to hear one another. Also, if a group member is sharing something important or painful, it can be very upsetting if this type of disclosure coincides with a burst of laughter or a blare of music from the adjoining area. Such an occurrence can often set off a burst of laughter in the group, especially from members who are feeling tense and anxious. Outbursts can be quite inap-

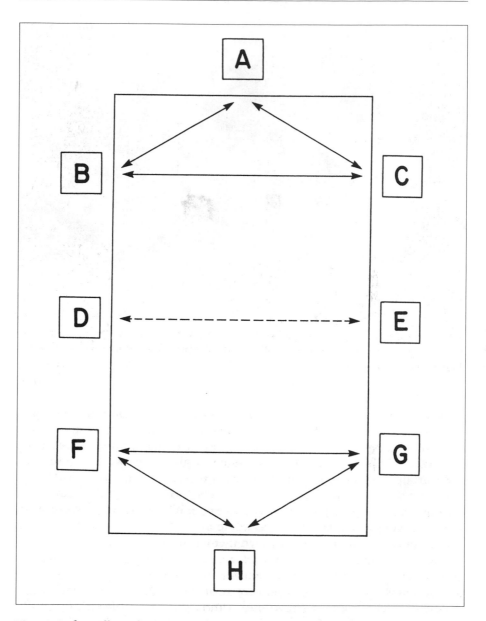

Figure 3–6.   Effect of seating configuration on communication patterns.

propriate in relation to the process going on in the group at the time. So, as much as possible, try to control the exterior environment so that it, as well as the environment in the room, is conducive to feelings of safety among members.

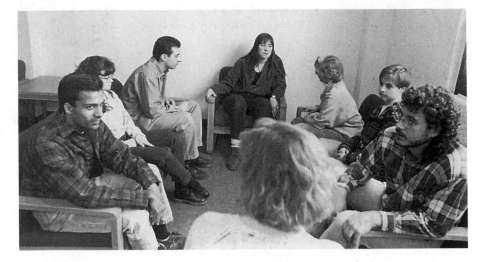

Figure 3–7. Interaction problems with poor seating arrangements.

Dress Dressing for a group does not really differ from the general re-quirements of dressing in good taste for the other aspects of a professional's work. Just as clients give messages to others by the way they dress, so do we as leaders give messages to them. Clothing can indicate attitudes, moods, personality characteristics, self-esteem, and emotional states. The way we dress can also affect our interactions with and influence on others. Brilhart (1974) warns, "For better or worse, we ignore the impact of our adornment in small groups at the peril of being less effective than desired" (p. 49).

Practically and socially one's dress should suit the activity of the session. If the group is going to be doing some exercises or is expected to work while sitting on the floor, then slacks are going to be more appropriate than a tight skirt. For a group outing to a restaurant or community event, appropriate at-tire for the time and place serves as a role model and reminder to clients to try and look their best because it is in their own best interest.

Whether you are male or female, as a leader you should avoid wearing clothing that has sexual connotations or promotes sensuality. Often clients are grappling with sexual problems or younger members are attempting to cope with identity issues. Provocative clothing in and of itself can be dis-turbing and the cause of increased anxiety.

Emotional Factors

General Mood The emotional climate of your group is going to fluctuate from session to session. Individual perceptions of the emotional climate will also vary from member to member. These differences are thought to reflect

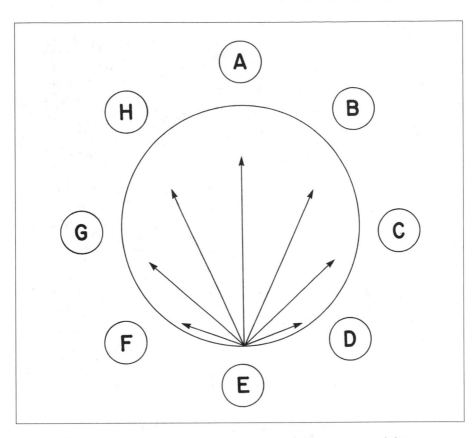

Figure 3–8.   A circle contributes to equalization of interactive possibilities.

the variance in members' interpersonal problems (Kivlighan & Angelone, 1992) which can change in degree and intensity over time. In a sense this means that a new group is formed each time it meets. One should never assume that because members are generally cooperative and cheerful one day, they will arrive in the same state the next day. Group members usually participate in a variety of programs so they will be having other experiences in addition to your group. Some of these experiences may be stressful and upsetting, some may be exhilarating and stimulating. When members come to group directly from these various other experiences, their moods will reflect a variety of feeling states as well. Because of this it may take some members longer to adjust and get into the group than it will others.

As mentioned, a group is basically a new entity at each session and therefore it is not possible to carry over the mood from one meeting to the next. It can even be difficult to pick up a discussion from where it left off at a previous session. It is a common occurrence for the most important issue of the session to be brought up just a few minutes before the group is scheduled to close. This can happen for a couple of reasons. The member may find it a difficult topic to discuss and so spends the group time getting up the courage to bring it up and, as time runs out, the pressure results in the member finally saying something. Or it could be that it is only by the end of the session that the member feels the emotional climate is safe enough to share the issue.

Such situations can present real dilemmas. Notwithstanding the problems with carryover, you might suggest that, since there is so little time left, the discussion be held over and brought up at the beginning of the next group. It is likely that in the interim the member will have an opportunity to discuss the issue elsewhere so it will no longer be of the same relevance to him or the group. If it is still an issue, you may find that he is reluctant to pursue it in the next group as the member may not sense the same emotional climate as previously. It is best not to pressure the member or belabor the point at such a time but rather to wait and see if he brings it up later when he feels more comfortable.

Your group will not always be in a good mood nor should they be. The purpose of most groups is to deal with problems and problem behaviors. For most people this is tough work and can be very painful. If the emotional climate is one of openness, caring, and sharing, then this will be felt as being supportive to members who may be struggling with themselves or with other stressful issues.

Mood of the Leader   It is important to realize that the leader, by virtue of her or his status, has the power to influence the emotional climate of the group (Edelwich & Brodsky, 1992). If you are enthusiastic, open, and caring, you have a better chance of eliciting these behaviors from your group members. If you are quiet, reserved, and cautious, it is most likely that group members will follow suit. New members especially look to you for clues and guidelines of what behaviors are acceptable and desired. Seldom will they ask but more often will be guided by the leader's behavior. Be aware of your own affect. Make sure your facial expression is congruent with your behavior; otherwise you can give group members double messages. Sometimes, we have facial expressions we are not aware of. This writer once worked with a student who always looked rather angry—even when she was feeling happy. Her constant dour facial expression caused the patients to be very wary of her and hence they found her unapproachable. Once she was made aware of this incongruency, she worked hard at changing her facial expression, with some positive results.

Mood of the Group   It is important to have an unremitting awareness of and sensitivity to the mood of the group. There is little that is more frustrating to group members than, when they on the whole, are feeling down or upset, to have the leader ignore their mood and proceed to be bright and enthusiastic. What is more likely to elevate the group's mood is for you to recognize and acknowledge the group's feelings by labeling what you sense—remark that "everyone seems a little down today" and encourage the members to discuss the situation. Sometimes, an incident has occurred during other programs or elsewhere in a center that is of concern to group members. Until the issue is dealt with, it is likely to be difficult and unproductive to proceed with the group task.

Mood of Individual Members   It is rare that you will find all group members in the same mood or frame of mind when they arrive for a meeting. Because they will all have had different experiences prior to your group, perhaps some positive and some negative, it is important for you to recognize these differences among the members (Kivlighan & Angelone, 1992). Some leaders find it productive to actually check out with each member how they are feeling at the beginning of the group. Others may find it more meaningful to comment on the moods of individual members as they sense them. For example, on noticing that a member is particularly quiet, you might say something like, "Mary, you seem unusually quiet today, is something bothering you?" or "John, you look rather down, are you feeling sad?" or "It's nice to see you smiling, Ann, are you feeling happy?" If an individual member is in a pronounced mood of sadness or happiness, it can affect the other members—a very depressed member can bring other members down. Also, an exuberant member can be irritating to other members if they are trying to cope with some heavy feelings. Dealing with such situations is addressed more thoroughly in Chapter 11.

INTERACTION

The importance of member-to-member interactions cannot be over emphasized as they involve members in and contribute to the group's process. As part of this process they help members learn and afford an opportunity for members to practice the skills of expressing themselves, supporting and relating to others, and resolving conflict (Ferencik, 1992). The frequency and types of communication among members in small groups are affected by many factors. One factor is the size of the group. The larger the group the more likelihood there is of having nonparticipating members (Nelson-Jones, 1992). Often individuals, even those who could be described as confident, are reluctant to speak out in a group, and they are even more reluctant to speak out if the group is large. On this point Heap (1977) concludes that as the size of the group increases, "fewer and fewer members say more and more, while more and more members say less and less" (p. 135). It should always be remembered that members of a counseling or therapeutic group may be feeling a certain degree of anxiety, which in and of itself can be inhibiting.

The number of staff that are present in a group can affect the types of interactions that occur. Naturally as the number of staff increases, so do the member-to-staff and staff-to-member communications. To encourage member-to-member interactions the ratio of staff to members should be considered and maintained at an appropriate level. The staff-to-member ratio can be a problem in clinical settings where teaching is a mandate and several students require group experience at the same time. This situation can be handled by having certain students observe the group through a one-way mirror, although this arrangement does not afford the students an opportunity to practice leadership skills. Another practice employed by some clinicians is to have the students sit in the room but outside the group. In the experience of this writer this latter method can be inhibiting and disruptive to the naturalness and effective functioning of the group.

For task groups a key factor that affects the frequency of interaction is the type of task in which the members are involved. Some activities, by their nature, require greater interaction among members than do others. Through the process of activity analysis the leader should be able to decide with some degree of certainty that, given this situation, activity A will elicit more interaction than activity B. Try to keep this important factor in mind whenever you are selecting a task for any group. Task analysis is discussed further in Chapter 13.

The development of active subgroups or dyads in a group can affect the level of participation by the remaining members in the group. Members are hesitant to break in on a conversation that is going on between only two or three members of the group and this very avoidance tends to perpetuate interactions exclusively among the subgroup or dyad. An intervention by the leader is sometimes required to bring about a more generalized and more inclusive discussion.

The more group members interact among themselves, the more likely the group is to grow and develop. It is also the case that the more members interact and get to know one another, the more likely they are to like one another and so feel inclined to further interaction (McLees, Margo, Waterman, & Beeber, 1992). As discussed in the section on environmental factors, the way in which the physical setting is arranged can greatly affect the level and areas of interaction. When members are seated so that they can clearly see one another, they are more likely to interact. It was also noted previously that the emotional climate is a major factor in enhancing or inhibiting the interaction level among members. Members who feel secure and accepted in the group are more likely to interact in a more meaningful way by expressing their thoughts and feelings or sharing their problems and concerns.

A critical factor, not to be overlooked, is that a great deal of the interaction occurring between and among members consists of nonverbal messages. Some believe that only 10 percent of any communication is verbal, and that 50 percent of the message is conveyed through the body and 40 percent through the voice (YWCA, 1991). These nonverbal messages are not only a part of the interaction process but they also can greatly affect the process. A member's smile may be enough support to encourage another member to speak, or, conversely, an unfriendly glance may be sufficient to deter a member from participating. Nonverbal messages are constantly being given and received by all members in the group as illustrated in Figure 3–9.

All the output messages of each member are being received as input by all the other members and each member will be affected by these nonverbal messages in different or similar ways. For example, if member A raises his voice when speaking, this may intimidate some members who will respond

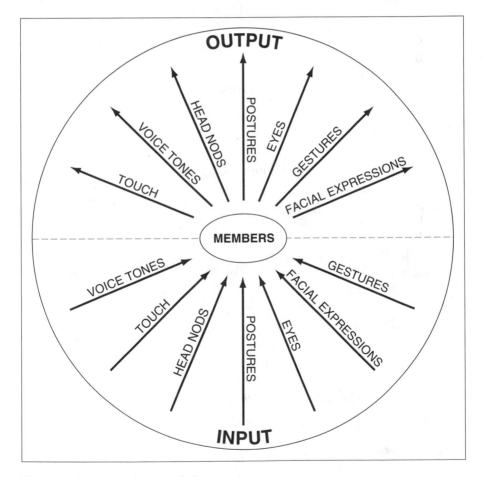

Figure 3–9. Flow of nonverbal messages.

by withdrawing, while other members may respond by becoming angry or argumentative. Member A may only be trying to make a benign point, but because of his raised voice the point can be lost as others react only to the tone of his voice. If member B is restless and constantly fidgeting, the other group members may tend to avoid interacting with him, thinking he may be feeling upset and not want to risk upsetting him further. On the other hand, when a member speaks and notices looks of interest and nods of agreement from others, he is likely to be encouraged to continue speaking and interacting.

Brilhart (1974) presents three concepts that he believes to be especially relevant to small group interaction. First, it is not possible to *not* communicate. Each member, at all times, is giving out messages and cues nonverbally. The way one sits, looks, moves or does not move, gestures, and speaks all tell others a great deal about oneself. Second, the meaning perceived from the nonverbal message is always received as being more significant than the meaning conveyed by the words. A member attempting to deny a disastrous social event may say, "It was great. Everything went well," but the flat tone of voice and his downcast eyes belie his statement and convey the real message.

These mixed messages occur frequently and require intervention, often by the leader, to help the sender realize that he is sending conflicting messages and to discover what he really means. This leads to the last concept— feelings, emotions, and attitudes are usually conveyed nonverbally. A difficult member may say he is glad to be in the group and certainly intends to participate, but his crossed arms, defiant look, and clipped words tell another story. A common situation is presented by the member who is visibly upset but who when questioned says, "There's nothing wrong, I'm fine." In such a case the leader must make a judgment as to whether she should pursue the issue with the member or if it would be better to let it pass for the moment.

The leader is, of course, also constantly giving out nonverbal messages that will affect the group members. Seeking feedback and checking to see if verbal messages have been received as intended will help you monitor and be sensitive to the nonverbal messages you are conveying.

INVOLVEMENT

The more members are involved in a group, the greater the probability of the group growing and developing. The degree to which members will become involved in a group is directly related to the degree of attractiveness the group holds for them. Members will be attracted to the group if they like the other members, the leader, or the activities; if they think the group can help them; or if they see others enjoying or benefiting from the group (MacKenzie, 1987). The more attractive the group is for members, the more the members will become absorbed and occupied with the group. In a therapy setting it is often more difficult to elicit a sense of involvement from the group members, because frequently they are required to attend the group as part of their treatment program.

As De Pree (1987) says "to give one's time doesn't always mean giving one's involvement" (p. 138). Because of this the members of a therapeutic group, at least initially, may be resistive and disinterested. It is therefore essential for you to exert every effort to present the group and the idea of attending the group in a positive way. Needless to say, the group will have to live up to any such assertions for the members to remain involved. Therefore the tasks, topics, and activities selected should be creative, interesting, and engaging.

Most leaders will be able to judge the degree of involvement of individual members by their attendance, their level of participation, and the degree of interest they show in the task or other members. If the members appear uninvolved or apathetic, it is important to assess the situation carefully to determine why the group is unattractive to the members. Involvement may be low due to lack of interest in the task, lack of obvious relevance of the task, the low energy level of the members, the monopolizing of input by one or two members, or an incompatible mix of member interests and personalities. Including the members in the decision making processes in the group as much as possible is a way to engage members, increase their feelings of competency, and therefore encourage involvement.

COHESION

Moos (1986) believes that the degree of cohesiveness present in a group is directly related to and partly determined by the degree of involvement felt by the members. Members who together choose to be actively involved in a group will experience a sense of "we-ness" and solidarity known as *cohesion*. This unity results from members sharing themselves, trying to understand others, accepting others, and allowing interest and caring for others to develop. Of significance is the fact that cohesion is more likely to develop when members adopt a here-and-now orientation rather than a there-and-then (past events) orientation (Slavin, 1993). Cohesion is seen as the sum of or the coming together of the feelings of attraction felt by all the members for the group. It is a feeling state that can be sensed when members like being together and like what they are doing. Braaten (1991) describes five "paired labels" that contribute to the development and demonstrate the presence of cohesion in a group: (1) attraction and bonding; (2) support and caring; (3) listening and empathy; (4) self-disclosure and feedback; and (5) process performance and goal attainment (p. 44).

Cohesion can be a strong and productive force in influencing the behavior and attitudes of group members and hence the overall group process (Budman, Soldz, Demby, Davis, & Merry, 1993). Members enjoy and feel comfortable in a cohesive environment and will behave in ways to maintain rather than disrupt such a state of togetherness. Rudestam (1982) says: "The more cohesive a group is, the more group control there is over the attitudes and actions of its members, the more conformity and commitment to group norms, and the greater acceptance of group values" (p. 19). A cohesive group has a climate of trust. This permits members to feel secure and be more open in sharing thoughts and feelings, including the giving and receiving of both positive and negative feedback. A trusting environment also fosters the expression of opposing views, ideas, and beliefs so that a more thorough examination of issues is possible.

A cohesive group is usually a productive and growing group, but there are times when the feelings of we-ness become too strong (Frank, 1992). This is evident when the members become closed to new members or new directions and invest their energies only in protecting the status quo. An intense feeling of unity, sometimes called a *group think* (Kurtz, 1992), can prevent members from disagreeing or behaving in any manner that could possibly produce conflict. Members become hesitant to give honest feedback if it is not positive. They may back away from personal problems or issues they see as potential areas of discomfort for any member. Such an environment prevents further growth or development of the group as an entity and of the members individually.

PRODUCTIVITY

Productivity, although somewhat different from the other group dimensions, is none the less an important aspect of any group. Members need to feel that the time they spend in the group is worthwhile, that it is productive for the group and for themselves personally. This is best accomplished if the members understand the goals or purpose of the group, if they are able to integrate their own goals into the goals or purposes of the group, and if they see the group moving toward accomplishing these ends (Gladding, 1991).

As mentioned in the section on stages of development, the production stage is the fourth phase and that is why a mature (ongoing) group is generally more productive than a young (beginning) group. A group may grapple with some or all of the other dimensions and phases before achieving the satisfaction of end productivity. The interdependent relationship between cohesiveness and productivity should be emphasized. It was noted in the previous section that a cohesive group is usually a productive group and the converse is also true: A productive group is usually a cohesive group. These two components of a group affect each other reciprocally and an increase in one tends to produce an increase in the other.

In counseling and therapy groups, productivity cannot be defined as clearly or easily as it can be in a straight task group. A task may be used in other groups but because it frequently serves as a catalyst, and not an end in itself, it would be the results of this catalytic effect that would be seen as productive or unproductive. This is an important reason to select the task with care.

SUMMARY

The importance of the effects of the environment on the process and functioning of a group cannot be overemphasized. Many of the points made in this chapter may appear to be based on common sense but it is surprising how many of them, through habituation or nonthinking, can be ignored. Leaders must remember that they themselves have participated in and are familiar with the processes of small groups, but for many of the group members it will be a first-time experience. What leaders know, understand, and expect is likely to be all new for the members. To allay some of the members' anxieties and fears, the leader should try to make the setting as comfortable, inviting, and conducive to well-being as possible.

There are five main factors that can affect the growth or development of a group: climate, interaction, involvement, cohesion, and productivity. The climatic factor encompasses both the physical and emotional aspects of the environment. Physical factors the leader should pay close attention to when planning or organizing a group are space, temperature, seating, configuration, sound, and dress.

It is the responsibility of the leader to make sure the room is of appropriate size, the seats are comfortable and arranged to encourage easy interaction, the room is neither too hot nor too cold, and that outside noise or disruption is avoided. Emotionally, the leader must be aware of her own mood during any given group just as she must be sensitive to the mood of the group as a whole and to each member individually. This awareness of mood is crucial to understanding the process that unfolds in each group.

Because a purpose of every group is to have members relate to one another, it is important to know what promotes and, conversely, what inhibits interaction. It is the role of the leader to monitor all interactions, both verbal and nonverbal, to ensure productive and positive outcomes.

The growth and development of a group is directly related to the involvement of the members, which in turn has a direct bearing on the degree of cohesiveness that will develop in the group. Both involvement and cohesion bring members closer together and are therefore desired factors in and of themselves as well as being factors that contribute to the overall productivity of the group.

Chapter 4

Goals and Norms

Before starting on a journey, we first
develop some idea of the destination.
— JOHN BRILHART

Everything we do in life, be it sleeping, working, or playing, is goal-directed behavior. When we sleep, we hope to be rested when we awake. For most people financial reward is a primary goal of work, although there are those who would say that enjoyment in work and a feeling of being productive is of more importance. Certainly enjoyment, fun, and pleasure are the basic goals of play.

Often we cannot achieve our goals alone, so we seek out others who can assist, are similarly involved, or who have the same goals. If we wish to play baseball, we join a baseball team. If we have a concern about an environmental issue, we may try to find others who share this concern and move toward organizing a group to lobby the government for some specific actions. In each case we become part of a goal-directed group and in each case there exist goals that the group as a whole identifies and goals that members of the group identify for themselves as their own goals. These are known as *group goals* and *individual goals.* For example, the baseball team we join may have the goal of winning the pennant as their group goal whereas an individual player's goal might be to hit a home run. Examining the concept of goals, Palazzolo (1981) identifies individual needs and group needs as well as individual goals and group goals, but notes the difficulty in differentiating between them. He defines *individual needs* as "forces within the individual, the existence of which is inferred through behavior directed toward the achievement of a goal" (p. 22).

To carry on with the baseball example, the individual's need may be to gain recognition or approval for performance from his father. He sees hitting a home run as a possible means of achieving this, so he or she directs his or her efforts, perhaps through constant batting practice, toward this goal.

Table 4–1 gives examples of individual needs, the type of group through which the individual might meet the need, and what the related individual

Table 4–1.   Relationship: Needs, Group Choices and Goals

Need	Group Choice	Goal
Companionship	Friendship group	Friendship
Love and affection	Marital dyads Family groups	Sexual and emotional support
Achievement	Occupational groups	Recognition and promotion
Knowledge	Educational groups	Diploma, degree, honors
Public recognition	Political groups	Elected or appointed office
Competition	Athletic teams	Winning
Aggression	Military service	Defeating the enemy, domination
Altruism	Social service groups Volunteer groups	Well-being of others, helping the under-privileged

Source: From C. S. Palazzolo (1981), *Small groups: An introduction* (p. 24). New York: Van Nostrand Reinhold. © 1981 by Litton Educational Publishing, Inc. Reprinted by permission of Wadsworth, Inc.

goal might be. Hopefully this helps to clarify the differences between individual needs and individual goals.

Group needs, as defined by Palazzolo (1981), are "forces which develop out of group affiliation, and which promote concerted activity directed toward the achievement of a goal acceptable to the group as a whole" (p. 22). An example reflecting this definition might be: Members of a community outreach facility become dissatisfied with the confinement and lack of variety in the schedule offered by the staff and propose ideas and methods for expanding and diversifying the overall program.

Due to the difficulties in differentiating between individual and group needs, the optimal situation is one where individual needs are similar enough and blend sufficiently to become the needs realized by the group as a whole. Noting this to be the most favorable case, Palazzolo (1981) then points out the possibility of other less favorable situations occurring in the relationship between individual and group needs. These situations can occur when:

1. The needs of individuals and those of the group are so incompatible that neither can be fulfilled.

2. The group may function in a way that realizes the group's needs but not those of the individual.
3. Some members may work only toward meeting their individual needs to the exclusion and detriment, if not the destruction, of the group as a whole.

Because needs, both group and individual, are seen as precursors to the establishment of goals, these tenets apply equally to the blending and integration of individual and group goals. If the needs of the individual members of the group are similar and compatible, they will integrate to become the group needs. In turn, these unified needs will facilitate and promote the group's successful functioning and attainment of its goals.

GOALS

Following from the discussion on needs, goals can be said to be the objectives established in order to satisfy needs. As defined by Tyson (1989) "a goal is an image of a future state of affairs towards which action is oriented" (p 106). It is that which is valued sufficiently by an individual or a group to motivate action toward its achievement (Johnson & Johnson, 1987).

As noted earlier, there are two main types of goals: group and individual. The latter are also referred to as personal goals. Important to the success of the group is for the needs of individual members to be compatible with the needs of the group, and it is equally important that the individual goals of members be congruent with the group goals. The motivation of members to achieve either group or individual goals is enhanced by their participation in the formulation of the goals. Tyson (1989) lists these other factors affecting the motivation of members to achieve a goal:

- How attractive or desirable it seems in terms of anticipated rewards for achieving it
- How likely it seems that it can be achieved
- Whether it was imposed from outside or group defined
- How challenging it is
- Whether members will be able to tell that it has been achieved (p. 107).

It should also be mentioned that both individuals and groups can and usually do have primary and secondary goals (Douglas, 1991). Your stated primary goal in joining a bridge club may be a desire to learn to play bridge, with your secondary goal being to make new friends. For someone else these goals could be reversed; they see the opportunity to join the club as an excellent way to make new friends, with learning to play bridge as secondary but also of value. If we follow along with this example to the actual bridge club meeting where these two members are present, we get an idea of what can happen when individual goals are different, even though they are considered to be compatible. Let us say you are the person whose primary goal is to learn to play bridge. During the game you are concentrating on trying to remember the rules, bids, and cards played. However, your partner or one of the opposing players, who joined the club to make new friends, keeps up a steady stream of personal questions as a way of getting to know you (or another player) better with the hopes of starting a new friendship.

The problems, quick to arise in such a situation, are obvious. You, and probably the remaining two players, will have difficulty concentrating, forget the bids made or which cards have been played, and are likely to become annoyed by all the questions and chatter. So the player whose goal was to make friends has instead irritated those present and as a result has possibly lost the opportunity or chance of obtaining his or her goal. Although a bridge foursome is a highly structured group with inherent rules and procedures, the same kind of conflicts and problems can arise in less structured groups where members have considerably different goals.

Group Goals

In most social or working groups there are individual goals, group goals, and tasks. Tasks are performed in order to accomplish the group's goals (Barker, Wahlers, Watson, & Kibler, 1991). In task-oriented groups the task is often only the medium around which the most important aspects of the group occur. It is true that tasks are carried out to accomplish goals, but in some instances they are not of great importance in and of themselves. In these cases the important things are the interactions, behaviors, feelings, roles—in fact, everything that occurs in the group in the process of doing the task. Completion of the task may not be of paramount importance. More is said about this in Chapter 13.

Establishing goals in counseling and therapy groups is an important aspect of the group but can be a difficult process. Many clients are not practiced or skilled in consciously defining goals in their everyday lives (Brown, 1992). They tend to proceed with work and play and generally living their life, but if they were to be asked, "What are your goals at this moment in your life?," they would more than likely be hard pressed to give a definite answer.

This lack of goals can, in fact, be part of the underlying problems that clients are experiencing: They have no clear, formulated goals to give their life meaning. Possible responses to the question might go something like these: "To do a good job," "To have a good time," or "To enjoy life." Similarly, vague, generalized goals are often noted by group members. Initially, if a member is asked to state his goals for being in the group, a probable answer would be, "To get better," or even, "I don't know. My doctor [counselor or therapist] just told me to come to the group."

In addition, there are those members who only see their goal in the group as a means of obtaining a desirable end result—"If I come to the group

I'll . . . be able to stay in school, . . . get discharged faster, . . . get points for a reward." Still others come to the group to be "done to" and their response goes something like this: "I'm going to get better here." It therefore falls to the leader to be facilitative in helping group members first, to, learn how to define goals, and then to define goals that are meaningful and appropriate for them as individuals. It has been suggested that performance improves when members participate in formulating their goals and then state them publicly (Steffan, 1990). These individual goals must be congruent with the overall goals of the group (Mitchell & Silver, 1990).

Leader Goals

Task groups most often have a theme that globally reflects the nature of the group and, by deduction, the nature of the goals of the group. A life-skills group is going to have, as an overall goal, one of helping members become more functional in coping with the demands and exigencies of day-to-day living. A self-awareness group focuses on increasing members' awareness of their own needs, feelings, attitudes, and behaviors. Clients are usually referred to such groups following an initial assessment. Results of the assessment should determine areas of both competence and difficulty for the client. Based on these strengths and weaknesses, and in consultation and discussion with the client, the counselor/therapist selects the type of group felt to be most beneficial for the client.

This is the stage at which the client, together with the practitioner, begins to establish his goals. The goals established at this time may be several and more global than specific. For example, "lack of self-confidence" may be a problem for the client as determined by the assessment process. The practitioner suggests and explains how an assertiveness training group could be useful in helping the client develop more self-confidence and so it is agreed that the client will attend the group.

As mentioned earlier, it is the role of the leader to facilitate and assist in the definition of goals by group members. In doing so the leader must always keep in mind that the individual goals defined by each member of the group must be compatible with those defined by the other members and also with those of the group as a whole: the group goals. It is also the responsibility of the leader to ensure that the members' goals are realistic and plausible in relation to any external restraints—the physical setting, the number of sessions available, or the expected length of the sessions (Nelson-Jones, 1992).

Individual Goals

When a person joins a counseling or therapeutic group, it is most likely to be a group that is ongoing and has been functioning for some time. Programs in community settings are more apt to run groups in a series of sessions, more like a course, and prospective members are then required to wait until the next course starts. In this case, where the first session is the beginning of the group for all, it is logical to use the first meeting or part of it as a time for members, in discussion with the leader and other members, to establish their individual goals for the sessions. However, in an ongoing group this opportunity for goal setting is not as available and can too easily be overlooked. It is frequently the case that the new member arrives, is welcomed to the group, introductions are made, the activities of the group are explained, and the group begins. The wise leader will take a little time at the outset to facilitate not only the integration of the new member but initiate the process of goal setting by the new member. The following ideas can work together:

1. Suggest that group members share one or more of their individual goals with the newcomer. This actually can be of benefit to the ongoing members as well as the new member. To state or restate their goals like this can be very helpful to present members by giving them the opportunity to clarify and reconfirm their own goals.
2. Members could be invited to share one thing they have learned from the sessions they have participated in. This too can be beneficial to ongoing members. Directed to think about it, some members will be surprised to realize just what they have (or have not) learned.
3. Ask the new member to "Tell us a little bit about yourself" and "Do you have any thoughts on what you would like to achieve or get out of this group?"
4. If the new member appears quite tense and ill at ease, it might be wiser to begin the group after introductions, suggesting that the new member might like to "see what goes on here." Later on in the session the new member can be encouraged to explore his problems, needs, and areas of difficulty. From and by these interactions, he can be helped to define goals to work toward while in the group.

Follow-up

It is important that time is taken periodically in a group session to evaluate the progress members are making toward the achievement of both the group and their individual goals. This can be accomplished by (1) the members sharing their own assessment of their progress, (2) group members giving each other feedback, and (3) the leader giving members feedback. At this point members may also wish to formulate some additional goals based on what they have experienced and learned from the group so far.

Some goals are very immediate and visible. For example, a very shy person may have as a goal that he will speak up voluntarily at least twice in each session. When the goal is this obvious, it is easy for success to be observed, which in turn makes it easy for other members to give encouraging feedback. Other goals are frequently abstract, although the more members can be urged to define their goals "operationally"—that is, specific in terms of observable behavior—the easier it is for them to experience a sense of achievement (Tyson, 1989). This is where the leader and other group members can be helpful. If a member (in an assertiveness training group) says, "I want to be able to stand up for myself more," he can be encouraged to explore with the other members the ways to behave if he were to "stand up" more often. This might draw comments like, "I would say what I want," "I'd say no (or yes) more often," or "I'd give my opinion." These are observable behaviors that can be counted and as such make better goals than the general statement of standing up for oneself. They are better because the behavior can be recognized by the individual, the group members, staff, and other clients, so the chances of receiving feedback are greater.

It should be understood that clients are to work on their goals both in and out of the group so any follow-up discussion would deal with both situations. The member's own report might be that on a certain occasion he was able to say, "I do not like the music being played so loud in the lounge." Feedback from group members might be that he is contributing ideas more often during lunch conversations, and feedback from the leader might indicate pleasure that the member is now more able to suggest or ask for things in group, like role-playing a specific situation.

GOALS VIS-À-VIS TASKS

Goal-directed behavior may involve participation by the group members in an appropriate and complementary task (Tyson, 1989). A *task* may be defined as "an act, or its result, that a small group is required, either by itself or someone else, to perform" (Barker, Wahlers, Watson, & Kibler, 1991, p. 37). Tasks differ widely from group to group. They vary from role-playing life situations, to solving puzzles, writing down what you like or do not like about something, reaching a consensus, or making up a monthly budget. Sometimes these tasks are confused with the goals of the group. In a consensus task, although the purpose may be to reach agreement on the correct order of the information, the goals for the group are varied: to work together cooperatively, to enable members to experience both leading and following while becoming aware of their style of participation, to allow members to experience both success and frustration, to see how the group makes decisions, and for the group, to assume and deal with the responsibility of completing the task. Completion of the task may or may not occur and depending on the goals of the group may or may not be important.

Another task could have real meaning for the group in and of itself and in such an instance differentiating between task and goal may be irrelevant. The overall goal of a cooking group may be to organize, prepare, and serve a meal. Accomplishing this goal will require many tasks: deciding on the menu, making up a shopping list, doing the shopping, dividing up preparation responsibilities, cooking, and serving the meal. These tasks are performed in order to achieve the overall goal, but they also have inherent goals. For example, in drawing up a menu the inherent goal is to formulate a meal plan that is balanced and includes all the appropriate items.

The most important issue around the relationship between goals and tasks is for the leader to be conscious of both at all times. Every group leader hopes that the group will embrace the task enthusiastically and that all members will become involved and work toward its completion. With certain tasks, though, it is all too easy for the leader to become involved with the task to the point of forgetting about the goals of individual members and even the overall purpose of the group. Frequently the leader will participate in the task as a means of modeling and to minimize the leadership role. In such instances it is critical that the leader achieve a balance between observing and facilitating the group process and participating in the task. Even after extensive experience in leading groups, there are times when the task, the discussion, or certain members will captivate the leader's interest so completely that the leadership role will be disregarded.

HIDDEN AGENDAS

Whenever individuals come together to interact, the interaction occurs on two levels. On the first level the interaction is conscious and its purpose is usually publicly stated. This purpose can be to accomplish a task, reach an objective, or to work on problems, and this is considered to be the public or surface agenda (Napier & Gershenfeld, 1989). But under this public knowledge of purpose are "aims which individual members hope to achieve for themselves . . . and to which they commit energy and behavior but which have never been made explicit to the group" (Douglas, 1991, p. 57). These covert aims and desires of the members are called *hidden agendas*.

It is not always easy to discern when hidden agendas are present and affecting a group. Tyson (1989) describes some behaviors and processes that can be observed and may be indicators of the presence of hidden agendas:

- Emotions overtaking logical thinking;
- Coalitions and cliques forming;
- Personal attacks, scapegoating, complaining, grumbling;
- Interruptions and over-talking;
- Ambivalence of opinion or commitment;
- Scattered, fragmented work procedures;
- Withdrawal into silence;
- Backing away from decisions at the last minute (p. 51).

Individual Hidden Agendas

Hidden agendas held by individuals may be conscious or unconscious and either way they can affect the overall functioning of the group (Andrews, 1992). It is this influence that should be recognized when considering hidden agendas as it can impede the group's progress. To deal with the tensions that are present at the beginning of a group, members tend to behave self-protectively while making advances toward other members in keeping with their personal needs for acceptance, recognition, and belonging.

If allowed to take its course, this process of probing and exploring by group members can be constructive in the dispersion of some hidden agendas. However, other needs such as the desire for power and the need to control others may not be aired and so remain present and unresolved (Tyson, 1989). For example, a group member who has a strong aversion to all persons in authority may test the leader to discover the degree of imposed authority, or as a protection, may try to wrest the position of authority from the leader. To do this the member may ask the leader about a certain rule that he knows has just been changed. This outward behavior appears straightforward and may even convey a message of wanting to be a "good client" by knowing and following the rules. However, when the leader responds with the old rule, the member corrects her, thus challenging the leader's position as the authority figure. The leader who recognizes this maneuver for what it is can, by conciliatory interaction with the member and the group, diffuse the attack while retaining her leadership role intact.

Other less hostile but still covert hidden agendas might be present in the member who attends the group only to receive "Brownie points" for personal gain, or the member who uses the group as a forum for displaying behaviors to impress a particular fellow member, perhaps someone of the opposite sex. These members, not committed to or interested in the purpose or value of the group, can be distracting and disruptive to the overall process and to the efforts of the other members.

Group Hidden Agendas

The group as a whole can also have hidden agendas. For example, if the group does not like the assigned task, their hidden agenda may be one of sabotage. Although this intent is never verbalized, members accept and even encourage undermining behaviors such as lack of cooperation, lack of participation, disruptive participation, or apathy. Another group may be resistant to disclosing feelings or engaging in personal sharing. In this case the group can defend against expectations of such interactions by sticking to superficial dialogue, joking, laughing, or going off the topic deliberately. In this way a group's hidden agenda can control the interactions and become established as an informal or implicit norm for the group.

Directly challenging a member or the group about harboring a hidden agenda is not likely to be productive. If the members who were constantly joking and laughing were asked if they were doing so to avoid intimacy, they are highly unlikely to answer yes. Rather, on examining her interpretation of their behavior, the leader might ask herself, "What does it mean?" "Are the members feeling pushed?" "Are the expectations for sharing too high?" "Is the process moving too fast for their comfort?" Based on hypothetical answers to these questions the leader may make modifications in leadership tactics, tasks, and style.

Leader Hidden Agendas

The leader may also have conscious or unconscious hidden agendas. On a conscious level the leader may plan a group in a specific way in order to facilitate desired behaviors in the group (Douglas, 1991). The plan might be to select a task that requires each group member to participate frequently if the task is to be completed. In choosing this particular activity the leader may be planning around one particular member of the group—the silent member. The idea is that through the use of this task the silent member will have to become involved in the group but can do so through a nonthreatening natural process.

On an unconscious level the hidden agenda of the leader may be to maintain the leadership role, with its attendant power and influence, at all costs. In another instance the leader may enforce the leadership role because she fears "what might happen" if she were to lose control of the group. This fear may be unfounded in terms of the group members' behaviors, but because it is beneath the leader's awareness, perhaps (in psychoanalytic terms) stemming from unresolved childhood issues of control, it continues to influence her leadership style. Behaviors displayed by a leader to maintain power and control could be: disregarding ideas and suggestions from members, disagreeing with members, invoking rules, and using sarcasm. On recognition of any of these behaviors in herself, the leader must try to analyze her feelings as objectively as possible and attempt to alter or modify her manner.

NORMS

All groups, social and therapeutic, formal and informal, have sets of standards that govern the way in which members' behaviors are judged. These standards are known as *norms*. Norms are formed through the acceptance or rejection of certain behaviors by a majority of the group members (McCollom, 1990) and are often associated with words such as "ought" and "should" (Tyson, 1989). Norms evolve in each and every group and are specific to that particular group (Borg & Bruce, 1991) although certainly several groups may have similar or the same norms. A behavior cannot be described as being intrinsically conforming or deviant. A behavior can only be deviant or conforming in relation to the norms of the group within which it occurs. A man who swears while sharing the bench with his fellow team players at a football game may not be considered deviant. He may be conforming to the way his team members express their frustrations and disappointments throughout the game. Given other settings, for example, with family or friends, this same man may express his frustrations without profanity. He is accepting and abiding by the social norms he feels are present in the two different situations.

According to Gladding (1991), it is through norms that "group members learn to regulate, evaluate, and co-ordinate their actions" (p. 199). The acceptance by individuals of being controlled by norms or adhering to norms is part of the socialization process that occurs as one experiences society as a whole. This learning is then extended to specific and smaller units of society. Individuals come to believe that conforming to the norms of the group is what is best for them and best for the group. If individuals are accepted as having a basic need to *belong* (Maslow, 1968), then this need becomes a strong motivator for them to behave in ways that will ensure their acceptability in any given group. By doing this they are accepting the norms of the group. Each group to which a person belongs will have different norms and each group will enforce adherence to these norms in different ways. Some groups will tolerate deviance from a particular norm or norms by certain individuals, whereas other groups require strict conformity from all.

Norms function as the rules of the game and assist in the smooth running of a group or unit. They are guidelines of behavior within which members can behave with some degree of confidence. They "function to regulate the performance of a group as an organized unit, keeping it on the course of its objectives" (Napier & Gershenfeld, 1989, pp. 117–18). The application of norms may vary depending on the status of the individual. By virtue of her role, the leader may be exempt from certain norms or a valued member may flaunt nonconforming behavior but because of the person's value to the group the behavior may be tolerated. This is not to say the behavior will necessarily be tolerated forever. The group may eventually realize that normative behavior is of more importance to the group than the value of the member, at which point pressure may be applied to the member to conform or to leave.

Norms touch on all aspects of our lives—how we express feelings, how we eat, and so on. Children internalize the behavior of parents and take on these behaviors as their own. Even the roles of parenting are internalized by children, which is why children who have been abused frequently grow up to become abusive parents. These are the norms they have been socialized to, and hence are those they adopt.

Explicit Norms

Norms can be divided into two categories: explicit and implicit, or formal and informal (Douglas, 1991). *Explicit or formal norms* are standards or guidelines that are clearly stated and of which all members are aware. Information concerning formal norms may be given to all new members as they join the group (e.g., "smoking is not allowed during group sessions," "No one is allowed to go out for coffee once the session has started"). Such explicit norms are usually formally established for the betterment of the group as a whole. They may be decided on by the group as a whole or by the leader alone. Frequently a norm established by the leader, such as, "All members must come to group on time," is embraced by the group members as they come to realize the disruptive results of members arriving late.

Implicit Norms

Implicit or informal norms are not formally stated but evolve from prior standards or behaviors brought by members to the group and which the members as a unit embrace. It is more difficult for an observer to ascertain what implicit norms are operating in a group than it is to discover the explicit norms. In describing a hospital management team, Susan Cohen (1990) describes two implicit norms that developed within the team and inhibited the productivity of the group. Decision making was hampered by the reluctance of team members (from adjacent departments) to openly state the needs and priorities of their individual departments. This norm prevented progress in the team's efforts to develop a hospitalwide service delivery model. Second, even though the presence of conflict was felt within the group, an implicit team norm prevented the expression of these feelings.

Implicit norms can cause intense pressure. The pressure comes from feeling impelled to be and act like others in the hopes of being accepted. Such norms are evident and especially strong throughout the adolescent and teenage years. All parents have experienced the protestation, "No one wears those!" or "No one does that!" in response to efforts to convince an adolescent to wear certain clothing or do certain things. The power and control of such norms should not be underestimated. A bright sixteen-year-old girl was drawn to a school group who were nonachievers, but as demonstrated by their laughter and high jinks, they appeared to have a great deal of fun. Because of her good marks they resisted her overtures of friendliness with taunts of "suck" and "browner." Six months later, when she was failing three of her courses, she was grudgingly given acceptance by the group.

The effect that norms have on a group is what must be evaluated to determine if the norms are good or bad. In one group the norm may be for members to share feelings openly including negative reactions to others, whereas in another group the norm may be to share feelings and reactions, but only if they are positive. The extent of conformity among members to the norm of sharing is often directly related to the level of cohesiveness in the group and this norm may become enhanced as the group progresses. In another instance members may see the group as a place to vent the frustrations they feel about the schedule or rules of the facility and at certain times this may be appropriate and constructive. However, if the griping continues and a norm—"the group is the place to complain"—is established, then other personal and more productive issues may be excluded or neglected.

Reacting to Norms

Four options are open to a group member from which to choose a way of handling an established group norm (Hare, 1976). If he agrees with and feels positive about the norm, the member is likely to conform and even strengthen the norm. Conformity is often rewarded with acceptance and approval. Should he disagree with the norm, believing it to be a poor standard for himself or the group, the member can try to convince the other group members that the norm should be changed. If these attempts fail, or if he decides against trying to make changes, the member has the option to ignore the norm and behave as he wishes. Ignoring an established norm of the group moves the individual into the role of a deviant and deviant behavior often elicits hostility, criticism, and even rejection from the rest of the group members (Tyson, 1989). A more definitive reaction, if the member finds he cannot abide by the standard, would be to leave the group. Summarizing, the four options are:

1. Conform to the norm.
2. Try to change the norm.
3. Remain deviant.
4. Leave the group.

The most successful way of changing established norms is through discussion. Frequently members are not aware that implicit norms are operating in the group. The superficial politeness that often characterizes interactions during a group's first meeting can evolve into a group norm if efforts are not made to move the group along to more meaningful exchanges. Members may demonstrate surprise, and perhaps some defensiveness, or disagreement when it is pointed out to them that they are relating in this manner. The ensuing discussion is likely to engage the members in more open and personal communication resulting in deeper engagement with each other. There are also occasions when merely making an observation of conforming behavior is sufficient to bring about change. Reactions of "I thought we were going to . . . ," or "How is it that everyone . . . ," will frequently lead to dissolution of unproductive norms or behaviors.

By role modeling and encouraging desired behavior the leader can impact on the norms of the group. For example, if she confronts a member who uses profane language with, "John, I don't like it when you swear," this gives a message to the members that swearing is not OK, at least not OK with the leader. By doing this the leader is not stating an explicit norm ("There will be no swearing in the group"), but rather is submitting an opinion on a specific behavior in hopes of preventing the behavior from becoming an accepted standard. In this way the leader can be instrumental in establishing norms. To carry this example further, at a later group session where a new member does use swear words, it is quite likely that he will be informed by another member that "swearing isn't allowed here." The leader can role model in less directive ways that can also impact on the norms of a group. By sharing and being open with feelings, both positive and negative, the leader conveys the message that sharing feelings is acceptable and perhaps expected.

The leader needs to closely observe and analyze the process in the group to reach an awareness of the norms that are in effect. If she feels they are inhibiting group progress, she should try to facilitate movement toward their dissolution. If the norms are felt to be positive and productive in nature, she will want to be reinforcing. Of most importance, though, is the awareness. Knowing what norms are operating contributes to the leader's understanding of the behaviors and actions of the group members.

SUMMARY

People are drawn to groups for various reasons one of which is that they discern the group as a place where they can respond to a felt need and act on it through the goals of the group. For example, people who have strong spiritual needs will be attracted to others who share their needs and by joining together they can delineate goals that will find avenues of expression based on these needs. Unfortunately, not all persons are able to recognize their needs, and even if they are, not all are able to satisfy them through goal setting. This is especially true of persons who are experiencing emotional problems. Because of this it frequently falls to the leader to assist the members of the group in recognizing their needs and, based on this knowledge, assist them in formulating appropriate goals.

The goals of some groups are obvious from the assigned designation such as a life-skills group. Before clients are referred to a designated group, however, their needs must be assessed by a counselor/therapist or team and a determination made that these needs may be met in this particular group. In other groups the goals are specifically formulated from the needs of the assembled members. Whichever is the case the group must be planned so that the goals will promote desired outcomes for the members. To do this, the mix of individual and group needs and individual and group goals must blend, and success comes from finding a compatible mix.

Success can also depend on the presence or absence of hidden agendas and the norms that are operating in the group. The latter fall into two categories, explicit and implicit, with the implicit being those that usually evolve within the group and can affect the process in either a positive or a negative way. Explicit norms are usually stated at the beginning of the group or as required. It is important for the leader to give consideration to hidden agendas and norms whenever observing or analyzing the process in a group.

Chapter 5

Membership

We're all in this together—by ourselves
— LILY TOMLIN

Counseling and therapy groups differ from societal groups. Indeed, by the very name the purpose of a therapy group is to be *therapeutic*—defined in the *New Lexicon Webster's Dictionary* (1987) as meaning "curative." *Funk and Wagnalls Standard College Dictionary* (1982) adds, "having healing qualities." The former definition is emphasized in Yalom's original work where he presents his "curative factors" but by 1985 he had changed the designation to "therapeutic factors." We would not expect a societal group to be "curative." Rather we would expect it to be enjoyable, fun, and perhaps informative. Taking the broadest sense of the word, though, we might join a social group, or perhaps a book club, as a means of "curing" our loneliness and in this sense the group could be said to be therapeutic. However, the main goal of most book clubs is a literary one, accomplished through presentations and discussions on books, not one of curing the loneliness of its members. In therapeutic groups the main goal is for the experience to remedy or alleviate members' problems and distress—in effect, to have a curative effect.

Counseling groups, on the other hand, are not so much curative as they are exploratory. They usually involve well-functioning individuals and focus on educational, vocational, social, or personal issues (Corey, 1990). The problems that members bring to counseling groups are often situation specific and may be temporary in nature. In the group, members are able and encouraged to explore their concerns in a climate conducive to personal growth and problem solving.

For both types of groups the organizing and initial formation of the group requires careful planning and thoughtful answers to some basic questions. In addition to answering those outlined in Figure 5–1, the leader needs to consider some other factors such as "What will the members do?," "How long will the sessions last?," "How big will the group be?," "Are there enough members?," "Are there too many members?," and so on. All are critical issues. Questions of size and composition along with membership roles are addressed in this chapter.

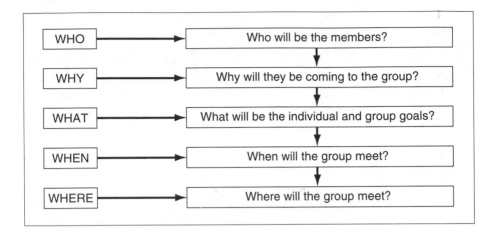

Figure 5–1.   Pregroup issues.

Source: Adapted from C. L. Knell and P. R. Corts, *Fundamentals of effective group communication.* New York: Macmillan, 1980. Used with permission.

SIZE

Size is an important consideration when forming any type of group. A desirable size for any group will depend on the age of the members, experience of the leaders, type of group, and types of presenting problems (Corey, 1990). The optimum number of members for a therapy group is thought to be five or six (Levine, 1979) and for a counseling group, no more than eight (Edelwich & Brodsky, 1992). It is important that every member has an opportunity to participate, and there is evidence to suggest that to achieve mutual interaction in a discussion group less than eight to ten people should be involved (Douglas, 1991). Investigations by Wheelan and McKeage (1993) indicate a marked decrease in participation, productivity, and the development of cohesion as the group size increased.

Shaffer and Galinsky (1989) note that groups of ten or more are likely to divide into two subgroups—one composed of the active group members and the other of the more passive members. While Levine believes that four is the minimum number for a group, Yalom (1983) suggests that even a group of three can occasionally function very successfully. Wide fluctuations in size are usually unavoidable and the number of persons available for a group often depends on factors outside the control of the leader. Most important, the appropriate number of members for any given group will depend on the purpose, structure, and capacities of the persons involved. Capacity even includes the confidence and skill of the leader (Nelson-Jones, 1992). Novice leaders may not feel comfortable attempting to lead a large group.

The size of the group will determine the extent to which interpersonal relationships and hence cohesiveness will develop among the members. Ten or more members may function productively in client self-government groups, social groups, or mutual-aid groups but one would not expect any depth of intimacy to develop in these groups (Geller, 1982; Luft, 1984). While Sampson and Marthas (1981) point out the increase in number and variety of resources in a larger membership, they also note the correlation between an increase in group size and a decrease in time for member participation.

An ongoing group can survive periodic low membership sessions since some degree of unity will have already been established. This may, however, result in the nature of the group changing due to the missing roles of the absent members. It is important that the leader expect and be sensitive to differences and changes in the group when members leave the group or are away, or when new members join. When such incidents occur, as will be discussed later under termination, the leader must be facilitative in helping the members adapt to changes in the group climate.

COMPOSITION

Membership of groups is determined in a variety of ways. In a facility where the team approach is used, the clients on each team may be included in a group led by staff from their particular team. A different strategy is to include clients, according to their diagnosis or level of functioning, in selective and representative groups (Ross, 1991). Membership in counseling or task groups usually depends on identified problems, level of functioning, and projected goals of the clients.

Whether the reference is to diagnosis, age, gender, problems, or level of functioning, there are discrepant views on the issue of homogeneity or heterogeneity of membership in groups (Gladding, 1991). For a group to "gel," Finlay (1993) believes that there should be some identification or commonality among the members. Donohue (1982) makes a case for the "identification group"—a group where membership is based on same age and gender. An identification group, she believes, gives members a feeling of "solidarity" that leaves them "with a feeling of relative comfort and security" (p. 5). Having had this positive experience, clients may be motivated to seek out a similar reference group as a means of support following discharge.

Hansen, Warner, and Smith (1980) believe that homogeneous groups operate at a more superficial level and are less successful in changing permanent behavior. However, these same authors credit homogeneous groups with being more cohesive, having better attendance, fewer conflicts, and faster relief of symptoms with evidence of mutual support. Based on the intrinsic value of homogeneity Ross (1991) presents a five-step format for groups of neurologically impaired individuals as she believes that they need additional structure and routine to promote response. Also based on the reasoning of homogeneity, Kaplan (1988) formulated what she named the Directive Group to meet the needs of acutely ill, minimally functioning individuals.

Sadock and Kaplan (1972) promote heterogeneous groups for several reasons. They believe having men and women interact together in the same group offers more options for discussion and presents a more normative situation—a microcosm of the real world. They also point out that drawing members from only one category of illness or age level limits the group's resources by restricting its access to a variety of behavioral patterns and ways of functioning. Bennis and Shepard (1978) support this view by noting that in a heterogeneous group younger members can learn from older members and vice-versa, disruptive members can benefit from feedback concerning their inappropriate behaviour, and those who are withdrawn can be drawn out by more active members. As multiculturalism continues to advance and groups become more heterogeneous in this respect "facilitators must be cognizant of the differences in personal characteristics between majority and minority members" (Kirchmeyer, 1993, p. 146). These differences can negatively affect the participation and performance levels of minorities in groups. Kirchmeyer found that the effective communication skills, assertiveness, and less expressed concern by majority members appeared to discourage participation by minority members. Also people from different cultures have different beliefs and interactive styles in handling conflict, intimacy, or negotiation.

R. C. Erickson (1986) argues that, given the constraints of the setting, heterogeneous groups may be the only option open to leaders on a short stay inpatient unit. In this setting he suggests the issue is not assigning clients to groups according to their needs, but rather adjusting the goals of the current groups to meet the needs of the members. Toothman (1978) suggests that while it may be best to exclude persons who are acutely psychotic, extremely hostile and aggressive, very impulsive or those with offensive mannerisms, he does recommend that membership should be representative of the general population. He also cautions that in all instances the selection or acceptance of members should reflect what the leader is able to tolerate or cope with. The reality of most situations is that the selection of members for any group is limited to the clients available and is influenced by their needs.

To be most effective, counselors and therapists should plan and organize their groups in response to the needs of their current client population. For example, if a therapist has several clients who have become dysfunctional through withdrawal and dependence, then she may establish a life-skills group. Similarly the therapist might choose some of these same clients along with other more diffident clients to form a group in assertiveness training. In other settings the unit or department may offer an assortment of task groups on an ongoing basis to which clients are referred as their problems and needs are determined. Another option for a department is to offer a basic group with various tasks to serve as an assessment group. On admission, all clients attend this group initially so that the therapist(s) can determine the clients' needs and then refer them to the appropriate theme groups.

ROLES

Throughout any group session each individual member functions in one or more roles, and these may change as the group progresses. It is important for the leader to have an understanding of the various roles carried out by group members in order to grasp the overall dynamics of the group as it unfolds. One way to do this is look at the behaviors and interactions of individual members. This enables one to determine the kinds of roles each member assumes in the group and the role in which they primarily function. Determining these roles gives the therapist important information about each member and how he interacts with others. This does not necessarily mean the members always behave in this role or manner outside of the group, but it is usually a good indicator of how they sometimes behave in their real-life groups such as family, work, or leisure.

Becoming aware of the various roles that members assume not only helps you in understanding the group process but enables you to be facilitative in increasing members' awareness of their behaviors and inherent ramifications. Say you have a member who appears quite involved in the group, speaks up frequently, and seems quite interested in the other members. Overall he is considered to be a "good participator." However, on closer observation of this member's input, you find that his interactions always have him in the role of questioner. Since this mode of interacting can be seen as a very effective way to keep the other members from getting to know him, it is important to determine what prompts him to keep the other members at a distance. By verbally making this observation (and the interpretation, if it seems to be appropriate) to the member, you can facilitate a discussion of this aspect of his participation in the group—and perhaps in his life in general.

Several authors have presented methods for analysis of group interaction (Bales, 1970) and functional member roles (Benne & Sheats, 1948; Dimock, 1985a). The classic functional member roles as laid down by Benne and Sheats (1948) have been utilized by many leaders, including this author. They delineate a variety of roles and are useful to the group observer in determining the manner of participation of the various group members. Because members usually confine themselves to a limited range of roles, the observer is able to formulate a defined image of each member's unique participation style. As feedback to members, this information can be useful in helping them become more flexible by changing or expanding their roles. The leader must also be aware of her assumption of these roles and through objective analysis or feedback from others define a personal style. From this analysis the leader too may see a need for more flexibility or more definitive changes.

Member roles are divided into three general categories: (1) group task roles, (2) group building and maintenance roles, and (3) individual roles. The roles are discussed in detail in the following sections.

Group Task Roles

Group task roles are those that aid the group in defining and carrying out the task or goals of the group. There are twelve roles that may be seen as the working roles of the group.

1. The *initiator–contributor* suggests or proposes new ideas to the group. These may take the form of new goals, suggested solutions to difficulties encountered by the group, or different ways of regarding the group problem. The initiator-contributor can also be regarded as the person who mobilizes the group through his or her contribution, either initially or when the group gets bogged down.

2. The *information seeker* seeks clarification of offered suggestions in terms of their factual certainty and looks for authoritative information and facts pertinent to the problem at hand.

3. The *opinion seeker* does not focus primarily on the facts of the case but asks for clarification of the values relevant to the group's undertaking or of those involved in suggestions made.

4. The *information giver* offers facts or pieces of information that are "authoritative," or relates personal experiences relevant to the group issue.

5. The *opinion giver* states beliefs or opinions concerning any suggestions made. He or she emphasizes a proposal of what should become the group's view of pertinent values, rather than the relevant facts of information.

6. The *elaborator* explains suggestions in terms of examples or expanded meanings, offers a rationale for suggestions previously made, and speculates on how an idea or suggestion would work out if adopted by the group.

7. The *coordinator* tries to clarify the relationships between various ideas and suggestions, attempts to pull ideas and suggestions together, and tries to coordinate the activities of the various members or subgroups.

8. The *orienter* summarizes what has occurred and then defines the progress of the group, points to departures from agreed-on aims or goals, and questions the direction of the group discussion.

9. The *evaluator–critic* assesses the accomplishments of the group in relation to some standard or set of standards that are relevant to the

group task. Thus this member may evaluate or question the "practicality," the "logic," or the "facts" of suggestions or of the manner of proceeding.

10. The *energizer* prods the group to action or decision, and attempts to stimulate or arouse the group to "greater" or "higher quality" activity.

11. The *procedural technician* is the handy person of the group and expedites group movement by performing routine tasks; for example, distributing materials, sharpening pencils, running audio-visuals, or rearranging the seating.

12. The *recorder* takes notes, makes lists, writes down suggestions, records group decisions, and generally serves as the "group memory."

Group Building and Maintenance Roles

Group members functioning in these roles are caring and oriented toward helping the group work well together. Their purpose is to build and maintain group-centered attitudes, behaviors, and activities. Descriptions of these seven roles follow:

1. The *encourager* praises, commends, agrees with, and accepts the contributions of others. He or she invites the participation of other members by indicating warmth, understanding, and acceptance of their ideas, suggestions, and views.

2. The *harmonizer* mediates differences between other members, attempts to reconcile disagreements, and relieves tension in conflict situations through minimizing differences, focusing on compatible points, joking, or "pouring oil on troubled water."

3. The *compromiser* operates from within a conflict in which her or his idea or position is involved. The member may offer compromise by yielding status, admitting errors, or by disciplining herself or himself to meet others half-way.

4. The *gatekeeper and expediter* attempts to keep communication channels open by encouraging or facilitating the participation of others. He or she may also monitor the length and number of contributions to accommodate participation by all members.

5. The *standard setter* presents standards for the group's functional achievement level or applies standards in evaluating the quality of group processes.

6. The *group observer and commentator* is vigilant of group process and feeds the accumulated data, along with interpretations, into the group's evaluation of its own procedures.

7. The *follower* goes along with the movement and activity of the group, functioning rather like an audience by more or less passively accepting the ideas and decisions of the others.

Individual Roles

These roles differ from the group-centered roles in that they are individual-centered roles. Within these seven roles members' concerns and interests are not centered on the good of the group as a whole but on meeting their own individual needs. The behaviors consistent with these roles are often disruptive to group progress because of antagonism to the group building and group maintenance roles. The seven roles are described here.

1. The *aggressor* may work in many ways. She or he may deflate the status of others; express disapproval of the values, acts, or feelings of others; attack the group as a whole; joke aggressively; take credit for the contributions of others; or generally try to put members down.

2. The *blocker* tends to be negativistic and stubbornly resistant, disagreeing and opposing without or beyond reason. He or she may dig in by attempting to maintain or bring back an issue after the group has rejected or bypassed it.

3. The *recognition seeker* uses various means to call attention to herself or himself. Whether through boasting, reporting on personal achievements, acting in unusual ways, or being overtalkative, the principal message is "pay attention to me."

4. The *playboy* makes a display of a lack of interest and involvement in the group's processes. This may take the form of cynicism, nonchalance, horseplay, and any other behaviors that convey the message, "I'm just along for the ride."

5. The *dominator* tries to assert authority or superiority in manipulating the group or certain members of the group. This domination may take the form of flattery, of asserting a superior status by having all the answers, giving directions authoritatively, and by not listening to or interrupting the contributions of others.

6. The *self-confessor* expresses personal feelings and problems to the exclusion of other types of input. He or she has difficulty functioning in the here-and-now with the group and tends to focus on the there-and-then.

7. The *arguer* has a strong need to disagree. He or she continues to present opposing views even when the rest of the members have reached agreement.

The group roles just presented will not be as clearly delineated in counseling and therapy groups as they are in a task or social group. This is because decisions are frequently required for the latter groups to proceed and progress, and thus a consensus of opinion may be needed or specific actions may be in order. This variety of activity and interaction allows and calls for more variety in roles than does a straight discussion. Because counselors and therapists frequently run task or task–discussion groups, becoming familiar with individual roles can be very helpful in observing and analyzing the process in the group. Certain roles, such as task roles, are likely to emerge more definitively during the task part of a group and decline during the discussion section. During a discussion group or the discussion part of a group, members are apt to function more in individual roles. Also, the leader may observe that some members participate actively in a task setting but participate minimally during discussions, especially if the discussion revolves around feelings. Observation of these behavior changes can form feedback to the members and may be the basis for members' increasing their self-awareness.

Benne and Sheats (1948) note that the combination and balance of member roles is a function of the group's stage of progress and development. In a newly formed group a leader is likely to observe more task roles, but as the group matures and members become familiar with one another and the purpose of the group, more group-centered roles will emerge. In therapeutic groups where members are grappling with personal problems and expecting help, they may try to meet their needs through functioning in more individual roles. On the other hand, if they are not ready to face their problems, members may avoid bringing attention to themselves by functioning in "follower" or "gatekeeper" roles. In this way, by focusing on the group and other members, they prevent notice of themselves and are likely to be acknowledged as agreeable group members. Because it is unwieldy to observe all 26 member roles when analyzing a group, it is useful to combine some and omit others that are very closely related. A suggested format is shown in Figure 5–2.

To use the observer's guide, the name of each group member is written in one of the columns across the top of the form. Each time members participate in the group a tickmark is put in the box under their name beside the role that most closely describes the context of their contribution. This is not an easy exercise because, as you are taking a second or two to evaluate the content of what a member said in order to record it, another member is often responding. Usually though, you can identify and record sufficient observations to obtain a profile of the group that can be useful in analyzing the group process. You may find it is too distracting to record on the observation form throughout the entire session. In this case it can still be helpful to use it for a portion of the group or for one or two time segments only—for example, the first and last 10-minute segments. This practice of completing a group profile is recommended for new leaders or experienced leaders working with a new group. It helps new leaders focus on the process of the group by examining the various roles that members play. It can also be useful in evaluating the progress or change in the functioning of individual members from session to session. (If possible, completion of a group profile is actually better carried out by an outside observer

OBSERVER'S GUIDE

MEMBERS

TASK ROLES					
Initiator/Contributor					
Information/Opinion Seeker					
Information/Opinion Giver					
Coordinator/Orientor					
Energizer					
MAINTENANCE ROLES					
Encourager/Supporter					
Harmonizer/Compromiser					
Gatekeeper/Expediter					
Follower					
INDIVIDUAL ROLES					
Blocker					
Recognition Seeker					
Dominator/Aggressor					
Out of Field/Argumentative					

Figure 5–2.   Member role observation form.

rather than by the leader.) As leaders gain experience, they become familiar enough with the roles to be able to identify the member roles without the form.

SUMMARY

Planning for a counseling or therapeutic group necessitates the same attention to detail that is required in the planning of any other type of group. Consideration must be given to and answers determined for who, why, what, when, and where questions. Size is an important factor and since the level of interaction among members is inversely related to number, it is suggested that the preferred membership number be between four and eight.

Based on the fact that we all live and work in a heterogeneous world (which is becoming more and more so) it is believed that heterogeneous groups offer varied experiences and more realistic environments for the members. Even groups that have been for the most part highly homogeneous in membership, such as a cooking group, are now considered appropriate for a combination of age groups from both sexes.

In a heterogeneous group, members will be found to function in a variety of roles, which can be categorized as task, individual, and group building and maintenance roles. To be familiar with the attitudes and behaviors of members as they carry out these roles and to have an understanding of how the different roles can affect the overall process is an important aspect of being an effective leader. Focusing on the presence or absence of certain roles can be very enlightening in group analysis. For example, the reason a group lacks cohesion and is not developing a sense of unity may be attributed in part to the finding that the members all tend to function only in individual roles. It is usually the case that having a mix of member roles results in a more productive and stimulating group. New members will bring new roles, feedback may alter roles, and reinforcement is likely to perpetuate roles.

Chapter 6

Leadership

*Empowerment is the collective effect
of leadership*
— WARREN BENNIS

People have been fascinated for centuries by the phenomenon of leadership. Bass (1981) reflects that "the ancient art" of studying leadership is evident in the classical literature of the Greeks, Egyptians, and Chinese. The literature abounds with descriptions, theories, research, and discussions of what is meant by leadership and what exactly constitutes a leader. The very breadth of the topic defies a single, short, concise definition, although Cunningham and Carol (1986) make the effort with "leadership is the exercise of influence" (p. 73).

Influential leaders from the past in the areas of politics, religion, the military, and sports have been recognized and discussed as a means to understanding the concept of leadership. Leadership has been examined as it pertains to the leading of a country, a movement, a political group, a profession, a faith, a corporation, a business, a social group, and the present focus, a counseling or therapeutic group. In discussing the role of the leader in any group, Johnson and Johnson (1987) expand on the concept of influence: "A leader may be defined as a group member who exerts more influence on other members than they exert on him" (p. 49). In keeping with the notion of influence, Sampson and Marthas (1981) describe a leader as a "person who is the most influential, who has the most power or the greatest ability to affect and alter the behavior of others" (p. 199).

In summary, leadership is assigned to or is assumed by persons who have exerted influence on others or are seen to have the ability to influence and thereby are viewed as potential leaders. In some instances, for example self-help groups, a person can be pressed into the role of leader by other participants who do not wish to take on the role but have a desire for the group to continue. In other cases persons may assume the leadership role because of their keen interest and involvement in a group's purpose or activities at a time when a leader is required. Whatever the case, any person who assumes a leadership role, be it of a Boy Scout troop, a volleyball team, or a political organization, is assuming a certain responsibility. Not always is the person aware of the degree of responsibility involved in the leadership role nor of the amount of attention required to carry out the role effectively.

THEORIES OF LEADERSHIP

Theories of leadership abound. Some theories focus on factors relevant to the emergence of leadership, while others address the characteristics and consequences of leadership. From the former focus two theories have been selected for discussion here: the trait theory and the times theory. Subsequent chapters explore characteristics and techniques of the leadership role.

Trait Theory

The initial efforts to define and identify leaders concentrated on personality traits and characteristics (Schultz, 1986). Proponents of the trait or "great man" theory believed that leaders were born not made, discovered not developed. The basis of this belief was that persons rising to positions of leadership were born with certain characteristics or traits that enabled them to achieve their status. Aristole is credited with being one of the earliest proponents of this theory of leadership, saying: "From the moment of their birth, some are marked for subjugation and others for command" (Johnson & Johnson, 1987, p. 40).

Countless investigative studies have been done to determine what personality characteristics are conducive to an effective leader role (Ellis & Cronshaw, 1992). Unfortunately (or fortunately, depending on your point of view!) the results were rarely found to agree on what were the essential characteristics. Most studies have examined the characteristics or traits of persons established as leaders in social milieus such as the military, political, and business domains. Many of the trait studies have looked at leadership retrospectively—that is, they have studied individuals who are in leadership positions and from analyzing their attributes have identified common personality characteristics. It was then assumed that these common characteristics were the basic inborn qualities that produced a successful leader. Results were inconclusive in that individual studies demonstrated a great variety of personality traits that correlated with successful leadership roles (Latham, 1987). Such studies also made the point that not all persons with the same traits prove to be successful leaders.

Following an extensive survey of the literature on personality factors associated with leadership, Stogdill (1969) concluded that leadership was not merely the possession of a combination of certain personality characteristics. He believed, rather, that the important factor in successful leadership was the acquisition of those particular personality characteristics that facilitated relating to and working with members of the group for the achievement of common goals. Conyne et al. (1990) describe these characteristics as valuing people, honesty, courage, self-awareness, flexibility, creativity, warmth, and a willingness to grow and change. Johnson and Johnson (1987) conclude: "Perhaps the safest conclusion to draw from the trait and personality studies of leadership is that individuals who have the energy, drive, self-confidence and determination to succeed will become leaders because they work hard to get the leadership positions" (p. 43).

Times Theory

Proponents of the times or situation theory propose that leadership is a function of the particular social situation. A person may emerge as a successful leader in one situation but he may not be able to transfer these skills or the leadership role to another situation (Dunn, Brown, & McGuigan, 1994). In exploring the prediction of behavior from observed attitudes and personality traits, Sherman and Fazio (1983) emphasize the role that the situation plays in such predictions. They point out that people are not necessarily consistent in their behaviors and that in order to predict behavior one must consider both the individual and the situation. The situational leader, or "roving leader" (De Pree, 1987), is believed to have attitudes and skills that are required and peculiar to given situations and will react in such situations by expressing these qualities behaviorally (Ellis & Cronshaw, 1992). These unique qualities of the leader are seen to match the unique needs of the other members present in the situation. For example, a basketball team may thrust the team member who is most knowledgeable about the rules and requirements of the game into the team captain or leadership role. However, it is obvious that this same knowledge and the attendant skills will not be of value to the person if he or she chooses to play hockey instead.

The times theory is similar to the great man theory in that it assumes that certain characteristics or traits are prerequisites to any leadership role. However, it differs in that the characteristics required for leadership to develop in a given situation at a given time and place are unique to that situation. The great man theory attempts to define personality traits that are inherent and conducive to the role of the leader in general, whereas the times theory avers that the person most likely to assume a leadership role in any specific situation is the person most able to meet the needs of those involved.

Theories and Practice

The literature on leadership primarily addresses the leadership role and the functions of leaders in public domains. As mentioned in Chapter 1, sociologists played the prominent roles in the earliest look at processes that affected the masses. By the late nineteenth century, however, sociologists were moving away from studying evolutionary change to studying directed change. Also at this time psychologists began to expand and broaden their study of the individual's involvement and interaction with others. Naturally evolving from interest in interactive issues came absorption with, and a plethora of investigations into the emergence and role of the leader in these collective situations. Resulting from and concurrent with these studies were the formulations of various concepts and theories of leadership.

Reflecting on organizational leadership and change, Bennis (1993) describes four competencies that he believes are present in and contribute to successful leaders:

- *Management of attention*—the ability to attract people because of a strong committment to an agenda, vision, or set of intentions.
- *Management of meaning*—the ability to integrate facts and ideas so that they make sense and have significance for others.
- *Management of trust*—the ability to not only portray reliability but to be reliable so that others know what you stand for.
- *Management of self*—the ability to recognize one's skills, use them effectively and learn from one's mistakes (pp. 78–83).

Both the great man theory and the times theory have relevance for professionals assuming leadership roles in small groups. Just as some persons assume the role of counselor or therapist with great skill and ease, so others assume the leadership role in small groups with the same degree of competence. The question is: Can the essential skills for leadership be acquired or must individuals be genetically endowed with them? It is the belief of this author that these skills can be learned and, although there are some basic skills required of all small group leaders, there are other skills that can be present in varying degrees with resultant successful leadership. We do not all have to be clones of a born leader!

Learning to lead a group can be likened to learning to play golf. When you are out on the course playing the game, you take with you a bag full of clubs each of which is different and each of which is used to make a different shot. The successful golfer knows what shot is needed in each situation and which club, given the individual golfer's skill and knowledge, is the best selection to make the shot. So it is with theories—you need to know about the different theories and then use clinical reasoning to decide which one is appropriate for use in any given situation.

In golf there are frequently situations where different golfers would use different clubs because of their unique skills and personal preferences but they can achieve the same end result and it doesn't mean that one is right and one is wrong. A variety of clubs are called for in golf; for example, a person does not putt with a driver but must use a putter. However, the number of clubs a golfer actually uses varies greatly. Some golfers carry very few and make do with what they have, others carry a bag full but still use only a few of them; other people carry a bag full and at one time or another use all of them. No matter how you personally make your selections it will improve your game if you have several clubs in your bag to choose from. And so it is with theories. You cannot do everthing from the stance of one theory. Being knowledgeable about and comfortable with the tenets of several different theories or frames of reference gives you a variety of options to choose from and to reason with in interpreting behaviors, in integrating information, and in making interventions.

THE LEADER

Most counselors and therapists must function in both individual and group settings. This means amalgamating the skills required in individual therapy/counseling with the skills required for effective leadership. In a group it is not enough to be purely the leader. One must function as a leader in a therapeutic or facilitative manner. Practitioners, and this refers to all health professionals who take on leadership roles in small groups, must have the education and training to function effectively in the role. As noted in this text, there is a body of knowledge as well as various skills and techniques that the leader must be cognizant of and proficient in. The degree of small group leadership training incorporated in the curricula of the various professions varies widely, but competency should be the goal of all (Gladding, 1991). Although health professionals function differently in their leadership roles than do leaders in the public domain, it is important to the understanding of their leadership role to first understand some basic tenets about leadership in general.

Just as the professions vary in their approaches to therapy, so will leadership styles among members of any one profession vary. Leadership style refers to the way in which a person takes on the role of leader in a group. This style usually evolves from the person's basic personality (Tollerud, Holling, & Dustin, 1992) and her or his typical manner of interacting with others. The style one assumes has an effect on the group and different styles evoke different processes and hence different outcomes. Sampson and Marthas (1981) believe there is a "self-fulfilling prophecy" inherent in the aspects and approach of a person's leadership style. Their premise is that "a particular leadership style gives rise to a particular membership style" (p 205). For example, a leader whose assessment of human nature is that clients need to be led is likely to adopt a leadership style of directing and being in charge. This assessment stands to be confirmed by the members as they wait for direction, becoming more dependent than independent.

Leadership styles can be viewed along a continuum, from the position of responsibility for the group being assumed primarily by the leader to that of responsibility being appropriated by the members (Edelwich & Brodsky,

1992). This continuum was outlined graphically by Tannenbaum and Schmidt (1958) and is adapted for presentation in Figure 6–1.

It is useful for leaders to periodically plot themselves on this continuum as a means of assessing their leadership style. A practitioner may not always utilize the same leadership style—the style may change in order to better respond to a situation or to a group's needs at a particular time. For example, with a newly formed group where the members have little idea of what is expected of them individually or of the group as a whole, the leader may decide it is appropriate and facilitative in this instance to be highly directive. With an ongoing group it may be the leader's decision to give the members more autonomy and to allow them to function as independently as possible.

This need for flexibility is seen as a major problem with the style approach to understanding leadership. Johnson and Johnson (1987) emphasize the need to adjust leadership style to the situation. In a situation where an urgent decision must be made, for example, an autocratic leadership style would be most effective. In a different situation where input from the group members is desired to ensure that the decision made will be implemented, a democratic style would be more appropriate. A laissez-faire

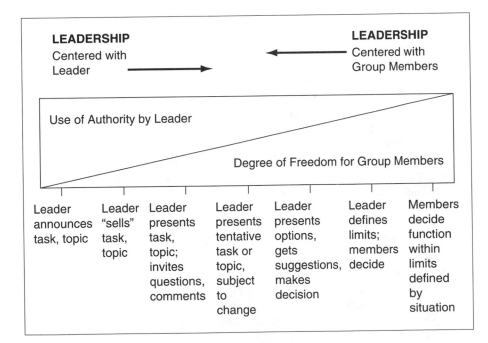

Figure 6–1.   Leadership continuum.

Source: Modified from R. Tannenbaum and W. H. Schmidt, How to choose a leadership pattern. *Harvard Business Review, 36,* 95, 1958. Used with permission.

leadership style might be best if the members are committed to a plan, have the resources they need, and the abilities to proceed with the project on their own.

The different leadership styles are described separately here only to help clarify the differences. The intent is not to imply that one is better than the others or that there are inherent "good" and "bad" components, but simply to show the variety of behaviors that are evident in and available to those in leadership roles. Each leader creates her own way of being in the role, by incorporating behaviors that feel the most comfortable and prove to be the most efficient. A sensitive leader combines whatever components of the three styles are needed to function effectively and carry out the leadership role at any given moment in the life of the group.

LEADERSHIP STYLES

The categories of leadership styles most often described in the literature are those defined in the classic studies by Lewin, Lippitt, and White (1939). These authors describe three styles: democratic—a member-centered problem-solving style, autocratic—a leader-centered decision-making style, and laissez-faire—neither a leader nor member-centered style.

Democratic Style

As mentioned, this style can best be described as a problem-solving style. A leader employing a democratic style attempts to create a safe environment within which group members feel free to express their views, thoughts, and feelings without fear of being rejected or put down. Members are encouraged to be themselves, to deal with their diversities through problem solving, and to move toward taking responsibility for the direction and functioning of the group. The process may be lengthy, as it requires time to ensure that all ideas are considered and discussed, differing opinions are worked out, and conflicts are resolved in an effort to accomplish the mutual goals. It is an active process directed at involving all members and as much as possible at meeting the needs of all members. De Pree's (1987) question pertaining to organizational leadership—"Would you rather work as part of an outstanding group or be part of a group of outstanding individuals?"—seems particularly relevant to a democratic leader. Some aspects of democratic style are noted in the following list. The characteristics of the three leadership styles, as presented here, have been taken in part from a concise summary offered by Verba (1961, pp. 208–209).

1. All policies are matters of group discussion and decision, encouraged and assisted by the leader.

2. Leaders:
   - Guide rather than direct a group
   - Are receptive to group members' suggestions
   - Leave most of the decision making to the group members
   - May offer suggestions or alternatives
3. Members are free to work with whomever they choose and the division of tasks is left up to the group.
4. The leader is objective or fact-minded when praising and criticizing and tries to be a regular group member in spirit without doing too much of the work.

Autocratic Style

In the continuum of leadership styles laid out in Figure 6–1, the autocratic style is found at the extreme left of the continuum and centers on the leader rather than on the members. Autocratic leaders are more likely to be found in the business or management world than in counseling or therapeutic groups. Studying organizational work teams, Cohen (1990) describes a hospital superintendent and her management group:

> Jean continues to be very directive in dealing with team members, and no one harbors any doubts about who is in charge. She structures all meetings, introduces the agenda, and forcefully argues her position. She has little difficulty making decisions and sometimes does so prior to receiving input from her managers. Most of the time, Jean makes the major decisions herself and thereby continues to keep the team as a whole from becoming fully empowered (p. 71).

Autocratic leaders like to have control and be in charge. They tend to *do to* group members rather than allow group members *to do* for themselves or *to do* in cooperation with the leader. According to Dimock (1985c), leaders whose style is to teach, direct, or dominate lessen the possibilities and opportunities for the group to grow and develop. Autocratic leaders often have a "I-know-best" attitude and do not encourage members to participate in the decision-making process but rather tend to make the decisions for the group. Members are frequently unaware of what is expected of them overall, of what the goals of the group are, or what is going to happen next. Partly by definition the autocratic leader is not interested in the personal goals of group members but rather operates from personally designed goals for the whole group. Alternative ideas are discouraged and discussion is kept to a minimum to prevent bonding between members. In short, the leader runs the show and members do what they are told or asked to do. This does not mean that such leaders are necessarily harsh or hostile. In fact, they can be very friendly as they persuade the group that they know what is best and what is the right way to do things. When members comply, the autocratic leader gives the individuals praise, which may appear generous but has the tendency to separate members and encourage competition for the leader's favor. In addition, group goals may be forgotten as members attempt to gain recognition from the leader.

All this may seem to imply that the autocratic leader is a "bad" leader. This is not necessarily the case as rarely does even an autocratic leader assume all of the behaviors listed above. It should also be mentioned that autocratic leaders often facilitate a very functional and productive group. As has been mentioned, there are times in a group's life when it is appropriate for the leader to assume a more authoritarian stance in order for the group to move forward. One example is when the members of the group are very low-functioning and are therefore unable to show initiative, make decisions, or assume responsibility. The main point to be cognizant of is that the person who tends to be autocratic in most daily interactions should be aware of the effects of carrying such personality traits over into the leadership role. The characteristics of an autocratic leader are:

1. All decisions and determination of policy are made by the leader.
2. Techniques and activity steps are directed by the leader one at a time so that future steps are always uncertain to a large degree.
3. The leader usually dictates the particular work task and work companion of each member.
4. The leader tends to be "personal" when praising and criticizing the work of each member, but remains aloof from active participation except when demonstrating.

Laissez-faire Style

The leader who adopts a laissez-faire style could best be described as a non-leader. As the French implies, this leader just "lets it be"—nondirectiveness lets whatever will happen in the group happen. Goals are not stated; the purpose of the group may not be clear; members are not discouraged or encouraged to participate; decisions are not made; and the leader, although very accepting, remains more or less removed from the whole process. There are times when untrained leaders fall into this style through lack of skill or knowledge of what to do. Other leaders adopt the style as a defense against telling others what to do or, as they perceive it, of being authoritarian. They believe the group members will rise to the occasion, take charge, and direct themselves.

In a group with high functioning members, this is probably what would occur with the possibility of quite productive outcomes. Unfortunately, what frequently occurs in such situations is that members flounder, feel frustrated, confused, and sometimes hostile, and generally are nonproductive. Occasionally a group member will emerge in a leadership role and attempt to organize the group. This can either offer the direction the group needs or, conversely, it can increase feelings of frustration in that a group member has to do the leaders's job.

In a counseling or therapy group, since such a situation can cause frustration and confusion, a total laissez-faire leadership style often only serves to increase the anxiety level of the members, causing them to withdraw and feel resentful of the group experience. One might argue that such a situation is a way to assess how members handle anxiety and to find out which members, if any, attempt to take charge. However, it is felt that the same information can be obtained by less stressful means, without the risk of clients being totally turned off to further group experiences.

A laissez-faire style of leadership, almost by definition, is not compatible with running a task group as the task itself lends some order and direction to the group. However, there are times when the leader will assign a task or a problem to the group with the instructions that they are to work on it on their own. This format encourages members to practice leadership, self-reliance, cooperation, and problem-solving and decision-making skills. The process, observed by the leader and experienced by the members, is then discussed so the overall dynamics can be clarified and integrated. Aspects of the laissez-faire style are:

1. Complete freedom for individual or group decision making, with a minimum of leader participation.
2. Materials are supplied by the leader, who makes it clear that she will only supply information if asked. The leader takes no part in work or discussion.
3. Complete nonparticipation of the leader in determining tasks and companions.
4. The leader makes infrequent comments on member activities unless questioned, and makes no attempt to appraise or regulate the course of events.

The three leadership styles are formally depicted in Figure 6–2. As can be seen, in the democratic style the leader's direct interaction is with the group and the group is responsible for decisions. This differs from the autocratic leader where there is no link between the group and decision making. With this style all information must be processed through the leader who, with little interaction or discussion, makes the decisions. The laissez-faire style represents very little involvement by the leader with either the group or the decision-making process, as the latter is primarily left to the group.

Two other styles of leadership, bureaucratic and diplomatic, are discussed by Burgoon, Heston, and McCroskey (1974). Although they pertain more to social groups than counseling or therapeutic groups, they are worth noting. The bureaucratic leader often has fixed rules to follow and as a result may be impersonal and rule-centered. She is interested in security, tends to avoid interacting with members, and demands loyalty. The leader's relationship with the members is more official than personal,

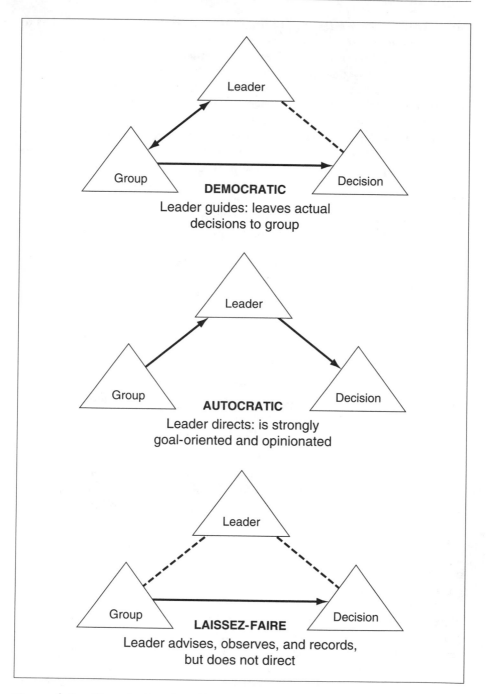

Figure 6–2.   Three basic styles of leadership.

which tends to precipitate apathy among group members. This style of leadership is similar to the "push" type of leadership delineated by Cooper and McGaugh (1969) and can be appropriate in some skills learning groups where certain required concepts need to be addressed (Perkins, 1992).

The diplomatic leader is described as Machiavellian because of the style's manipulative characteristics. The leader looks for personal gain through this leadership role and uses various tactics to achieve the desired ends. Although at times the manner of engaging the members may appear democratic, there is usually an underlying personal motivation.

Combination of Styles

Most group leaders operate primarily from one leadership style, which has as its basis the leader's own personality traits. A person of action who likes to get things done quickly and who has strong opinions about how things should be is more likely to adopt aspects of an autocratic leadership style than is a person who is more easygoing. A person who enjoys interacting and listening to the ideas of others, joining in a problem-solving process, and being part of a discussion is prone to be a more democratic leader. An aversion to authority of any kind and a strong belief in the autonomy and rights of the individual are characteristics that would lead a person toward a laissez-faire style. As can be seen in examining these traits, positive aspects can be found in each, which can be used productively in combination.

Let us examine the situation where you, the leader, are beginning your first session with a new group of clients. You have chosen a consensus task as the activity for the session. Initially you introduce yourself and suggest, depending on whether members know each one another or not, that the members also introduce themselves (autocratic). You might then ask if any members have any questions or anything they want to say before you begin the activity (democratic). You then describe the task, state the rules, explain how it is to be done, and give a time limit (autocratic). At this point you would again ask if there are any questions (democratic). During the task you might withdraw from participation and let the group function entirely on its own, even responding to members' clarifying questions with: "What do you think?" or "It's up to you" (laissez-faire). At the end of the stated time you terminate the task (autocratic) and move the group into a discussion of what happened during the activity and how members felt about the experience (democratic). Combining approaches in this way makes for a diverse and interesting leader. It can also be quite productive because group members feel some autonomy but are prodded to keep moving.

Having a clear understanding of the differences in the three leadership styles can be helpful in determining your own style. It can be informative to evaluate your personal characteristics and then relate and compare them to the leadership characteristics. As an example, you may realize that you are quite extroverted and a rather high-powered type of person. You like to make decisions and get things done. Knowing this you may conclude that your most natural way of operating in any group is to tend to take charge, organize, and prod members to action. You may conclude that your personality appears to embrace both democratic and autocratic traits but few that could be considered laissez-faire.

An awareness of the styles can also add to your repertoire of leadership behaviors by stimulating alternative actions. Say a group is working intently on a problem-solving task but five or ten minutes into the task, member A, appearing distressed, makes the following statement: "No one will listen to me." At this point in the group it is important to set aside the task temporarily and facilitate a discussion of member A's feelings. It is even possible that the task may be completely abandoned for that session in favor of continuing what has evolved into a productive discussion. For some leaders it is difficult to be this flexible. They feel a need to have the task completed and therefore will defer such a discussion or ignore the member's input until the task is finished. By the end of the task, however, the moment may be lost and member A or other group members may be resistant to discussing the issue. It is more difficult for members to recall feelings than to deal with them in the here and now. Discussing an issue in retrospect can lapse into a dialogue of, "You said," "No I didn't," "Yes you did"—the sort of situation that is obviously unproductive. On the other hand, if the discussion starts to meander off the topic or is resolved to what you believe to be (on checking) member A's and the group's satisfaction, then it is a good time to direct the members back to the task.

EFFECT OF LEADERSHIP STYLE ON GROUP MEMBERS

The behavior or style of the leader will have a direct affect on the behavior of group members (Sampson & Marthas, 1981). This is particularly true if the leader functions exclusively within one style of leadership. The behavior of group members as consequences of leadership style is known as membership style, and these styles are presented in the following lists, which are based in part on those Sampson and Marthas (1981) discuss.

Democratic Style

1. Members are enthusiastic about the task or activity of the group, displaying a high degree of participation and involvement.
2. Members are motivated to complete the task and experience satisfaction from being part of a successful effort.
3. There is a strong sense of unity or we-ness among group members as they cooperate and work together. Members are accepting and caring of one another.

4. Members feel good about their own participation and encourage it in others.
5. Members display initiative and learn to assume responsibility for the functioning and progress of the group.

Autocratic Style

1. Members will be compliant in doing the task but may show little enthusiasm. Participation or involvement may appear forced or stilted.
2. Members can be productive in working on the task but feelings of satisfaction are absent due to resentments and anger toward the leader.
3. Cooperation is low, and members may be irritable and blaming with one another.
4. Participation by members is dependent on prodding from the leader.
5. Members resist accepting responsibility, display little initiative, and are apathetic toward what happens in or to the group.

Laissez-faire Style

1. Members are confused and frustrated with the task due to lack of direction.
2. Productivity is low. Efforts at completing the task may be sloppy and inefficient.
3. Members are not unified and display little interest in working together.
4. Participation is uneven and unrelated to the participation of others.
5. Due to the confusion and frustration experienced by members with the purpose of the group, they tend to absolve themselves of responsibility for what happens.

It should be recognized that the member behaviors described here represent reactive responses to the leadership styles in their most classic and pure forms. Rarely does a leader perform "classically." Therefore these behaviors are not likely to be as definitive as described here and are likely to be observed in combination.

Observing the behaviors of group members, especially over time, can sometimes be cause for an analysis of your behaviors as a leader. If approached with a receptive mind, this can be an enlightening process and may provoke you to adapt or make some definitive changes in your approach. Self-evaluations should be frequent and ongoing (and not only when there are problems) to prevent repetition, rigidity, and stagnation.

SUMMARY

Formulating your leadership style is a very personal and individual process. Although new behaviors can and should be learned, attempting to function at complete odds with your basic personality set is unrealistic. Success comes when you can effectively incorporate your personal characteristics into the many facets and functions that form the composite of a leader's role. In this role you must direct, facilitate, observe, analyze, participate, listen, respond, and organize, and remember that you are usually seen as an expert. A mix of personal characteristics (the great man theory) and the situation (the times theory) will contribute to your success in these endeavors.

Although, the three leadership styles—democratic, autocratic, and laissez-faire—are presented separately, it is suggested that leaders incorporate those behaviors from each style that they feel most comfortable with and which prove to be most productive at any given time in a particular group session. In a similar manner to selecting methods and techniques from various theoretical approaches so do you select behavior from the different leadership styles. In general, you may adopt more behaviors from one style than from the others, but it is wise to be flexible and eclectic in your overall approach. It is important to keep in mind that your leadership style will have a direct influence on the behavior of the group members. It is a responsible and exciting role that is best carried out with sensitivity. Specific leadership skills and techniques are covered in the following chapters.

Chapter 7

Leadership Attributes

*The most effective leader is one who
can create the conditions by which he
will actually lose the leadership.*
— CARL ROGERS

One of the expectations of counseling and therapeutic groups is that the members will be involved in ongoing self-evaluation to facilitate change in themselves. Leaders should be involved in the same process. A group leader learns from each group experience, as do the members of the group, and consequently both are in a constant state of change. The leader needs to practice what all practitioners preach—recognizing negative and nonproductive behaviors is the first step toward positive change. Following each group session the leader will benefit from engaging in a self-analysis as well as an analysis of the group process. Self-analysis should focus on the feelings, thoughts, and behaviors experienced and displayed during the session. The following attributes of leadership can serve as useful referents in guiding one's self-analysis.

An inherent difficulty in delineating the critical attributes of a leader is that educators and researchers do not agree on what differentiates an effective leader from an ineffective one (Morganett, 1990). A secondary difficulty relates to the wide variety of attributes and characteristics that are thought to contribute to effective leadership. However, it appears that most of the attributes and skills that do contribute to effective leadership are the same ones that make a counselor or therapist effective in one-to-one interactions (Borg & Bruce, 1991; Conyne, Harvill, Morganett, Morran, & Hulse-Killacky, 1990). In addition, the individual's personality, the purpose of the group, and the nature of the members all must be taken into consideration when identifying desired characteristics. The attributes selected for inclusion here are thought to be representative of basic qualities displayed by effective leaders.

SELF-CONFIDENCE

In any endeavor we function more productively if we have confidence in what we are doing. Corey, Corey, Callanan, and Russell (1992) describe the most effective counselors as those who feel like "winners." Group members will be quick to pick up on lack of confidence in a leader and this may cause them to feel uneasy and wary of getting involved in the group. It is scary to take personal risks if you do not feel confident that the person in charge is capable and dependable. So a certain level of self-confidence demonstrated by the leader is necessary to inspire confidence in the group members (Kottler, 1983). By showing self-assurance, enthusiasm, and comfort in the situation you are more able to facilitate member participation and hence a productive group experience for all. Members' perceptions of an effective helper are formed from various indicators, one being "dynamism," which encompasses self-confidence and forcefulness.

Research by Goldstein and Myers (1986) demonstrated that people are more attracted to high-status helpers or persons perceived to be experts than to those perceived to be lower-status helpers. Of four variables selected by Schultz (1986) as predictors of emergent leadership, "self-assured" was the only one related to personal style. The three other variables, "formulates goals," "gives directions," and "summarizes" were all communicative functions.

Naturally, one gains self-confidence in the leadership role with experience, but even as a novice leader it is important to impart the message of capability. The old adage, "you are what you feel," holds true. If you present in a positive manner, called "performance self-esteem" by Stake (1983), and believe you are competent to run a productive group, then it is very likely you will have a productive group. Kottler (1983) emphasizes this need for a "strong sense of mission" in the leader. To introduce a task or activity with the comment, "This experience can be very helpful" will produce a more positive response from the group members than will the hesitant, "This might be useful, but I'm not sure."

In the same way members do, the leader takes her own fears, needs, and anxieties into the group; she wonders, "Will the group be successful?" and worries, "Am I ready for this?" However, if the leader is able to move beyond these questions from within to "hearing" these same questions in the group members, she will demonstrate sensitivity, awareness, and understanding. By doing this a leader will achieve a sense of mastery over personal anxieties, function more effectively, and present an aura of competence. Using each group as a learning experience will gradually but consistently build self confidence in the leadership role.

RESPONSIBILITY

This attribute, which embodies dependability, trustworthiness, and reliability, is an important one but a difficult one to explain. A leader can be seen to have dual responsibilities, one to the group and one to herself as a professional. The leader, often the only staff member in the group, must assume full responsibility for handling the "happenings" in the group. Members of the group need to feel safe and know that they can depend on the leader to ensure their safety by having their best interests at heart. There must be trust that the leader will behave responsibly toward all members.

Trotzer (1977) describes leader responsibility as being on a continuum. At one extreme the leader assumes full responsibility for all the "interactions and impact of the group," while at the other extreme, the responsibility is totally invested in the group, including the leader as an equal partner (p. 91). Most leaders operate from the *middle* of the *continuum*, giving and taking responsibility in response to the needs and level of functioning of the group. Frequently the degree to which responsibility is assumed reflects the developmental level of the group. When the group is in a dependent stage, the leader may accept more responsibility which is then gradually given over to the group as it demonstrates more independence. This transition could even occur over the course of one session.

Sharing responsibilities at times can be part of the goals and functions of the group. During a task or activity the leader may encourage members to accept responsibility by asking, "Who would like to keep the list?" or "Who will be responsible for announcing the time slots?" Responsibilities can extend outside the group: "Would someone set up the chairs for the next session?" sometimes the group may be given total responsibility for organizing the task or activity for a session.

Trust is an issue in terms of confidentiality. The leader must be honest and inform the members what the limits are for information remaining confidential within the group. These limits will vary greatly from one setting to another. A trustworthy leader does not tell a member she will keep certain information confidential but then report the information to colleagues. However, if working in a team, a leader also has a responsibility to colleagues and must tread this line with care. To be responsible to both team members and group members it is best to be up front with the latter by telling them that what goes on in any group session is usually reported back to the team. Explain the importance of all team members having the information in order to optimize overall treatment and goal planning. By explaining this to the group members, they then know where they stand in terms of confidentiality and thus can choose what they wish to share in the group.

As for reliability and dependability, group members prefer a leader whom they can rely on to behave in a consistent manner from one session to another. They like a leader who is dependable, who arrives on time, who makes sure a suitable meeting room is available, and who has given some forethought to the session such as having a task prepared or the required materials available for a planned activity.

ATTENDING AND LISTENING

To *attend* is to truly focus on the other person and to *listen* is to hear what is being said. Burnard (1992) believes that these two activities are the most important aspects of any practitioner's work. Although to some attending and listening may appear to be leadership techniques rather than attributes, they are included here because of their importance as personal characteristics. When asked why they joined a helping profession, counselors and therapists often reply, "Well, I always have been a good listener." People who are good listeners by nature tend to make good group leaders. However, if you do not count listening or attending among your main strengths, do not despair for they are skills that can be acquired through practice and perseverance.

The leader role is an exacting one as you must attend or be "tuned in" to all members of the group for the entire session. Sound exhausting? It can be. As a preparatory measure to this demanding experience it is energizing to "psych" yourself up to focus and listen before entering the session. Being tuned in means not only listening to what each member says but listening to how they say what they say. It also means attending to all the nonverbal messages members may be conveying. Frequently the latter are of more consequence than the former. Lakin (1983) recognizes that the demands of attending and listening to all the verbal and nonverbal communications occurring simultaneously among the group members is a major source of stress for group leaders.

The leader must listen very carefully and really hear what is being said in order to connect with group members. Another aspect of the leader's role is to encourage this listening behavior in others in the group to facilitate connections between the members. It is this linking that spawns the growth of trust, a condition crucial to the growth and development of a group. By listening and attending to members' responses a leader can tell if the members are actually listening to one another. The importance of their doing so can be emphasized by statements such as: "From what you replied I'm not sure you really heard what M. said," "What did you hear M. say?," or "Can you repeat what M. just said?" Sometimes what you hear and what you see do not seem to be congruent. For example, a member may be telling you how happy he is and how well things are going for him, while all the time he is speaking he is looking anything but happy. In this instance attending gives you information that differs from what you hear. To deal with the inconsistency you might say something like, "What I heard you say is . . . but it doesn't seem to fit with the sad look on your face." From these or similar interventions members receive the message that not only are you interested in what they have to say but also whether what they say is correctly understood by the other members.

There are many ways that both leaders and members demonstrate a lack of listening and/or attending:

- Lack of eye contact
- Interrupting
- Thinking of what to say next
- Talking too much
- Being off-topic
- Hearing what you want to hear

Effective listening requires concentration. It is better to listen and then take a few seconds to consider what a member has said before you respond than to be thinking of your response while someone is speaking. After all, you will not know what has been said until it has been said!

Besides actually hearing what group members have to say there are three other important functions of a group leader as a listener (Sampson & Marthas, 1981). First the "listening" leader assures members that there will be someone to hear them if and when they speak. Some members are afraid to speak out in group for fear that no one will listen or respond to them. When this occurs, an attending leader notices this omission and responds appropriately. The second function is one of modeling. The attending, listening leader is a role model in these behaviors for the members. When members observe the leader listening attentively and being responsive to group members, they can see opportunities for themselves to behave in similar ways. Finally when members realize that others are listening carefully, and trying to understand what they have to say, they are likely to sharpen their thinking and their ideas to warrant the concern of the others. The actual content of what group members say can generate many feelings, thoughts, and behaviors in the leader as well as the other members.

To assist in being prepared for such reactions Barker, Wahlers, Watson, and Kibler (1991, pp. 78–79)) list five listening pitfalls to avoid in a group:

1. Getting overstimulated or emotionally involved
2. Preparing to answer questions before fully understanding them
3. Tolerating or failing to adjust to distractions
4. Allowing emotionally laden words to interfere with listening

5. Permitting personal prejudices or deep-seated convictions to impair comprehension or understanding

Listening and attending are important aspects of client-centered practice and are discussed further in Chapter 9.

OBJECTIVITY

As in all counseling and therapeutic roles, it is imperative that the group leader maintain a firm sense of objectivity. Rogers (1961) describes an "as if" quality in defining empathy that can be related to objectivity. He believes that individuals who respond as if they were the other person without losing their personal identity can be empathic while still retaining their objectivity. A leader must be able to think clearly and maintain an objective awareness of all the members even when under pressure. To become personally immersed in the issues or problems of one member of the group is to be out of touch with the others. In addition, to experience this degree of subjective involvement is draining and depletes the energy required to deal with the other group members or the day's routine that follows. As leader, you can be empathic but remain aware that the problem belongs to the other person and not to you. Leaders must constantly monitor their own feelings and responses to ensure their objectivity. Indicators of nonobjective behaviors are: (1) getting caught up in the content and forgetting about the process of the group, (2) experiencing overwhelming emotions, (3) assuming the roles of advice giver and problem solver, and (4) arguing.

An integral part of being objective is the ability to recognize the presence of transference and countertransference among your members and within yourself. *Transference* refers to the stimulation and emergence of suppressed or repressed feelings in a group member as a result of interacting with the leader or another group member (Sklare, Keener, & Mas, 1990). As an example, a member may react angrily toward the leader because for him she stands for a significant person from his past, perhaps an authoritative or domineering mother. Because these experiences and attitudes differ for each member the reactions of the members to you will also be varied. It can be confusing to have some members react very positively to your participation while others seem quite resistive and negative. It is important to help your members recognize any distorted perceptions they may have, such as your being all-knowing or your being vindictive, and to help them work through the feelings toward you that have been engendered by these distortions.

It can be more difficult to deal with countertransference. Because these feelings and reactions occur within you, the leader, a great deal of self-awareness is required for you to recognize the dynamics that are taking place (Smith, 1990). It is only too easy to be responsive to positives and accept accolades while becoming defensive or parental in response to negatives or disagreement. The key is to try to maintain a critical awareness and sensitivity to all that is happening both with your group members and within yourself.

GENUINENESS

To be genuine implies that what you do and say is congruent with what is going on inside of you (Raskin & Rogers, 1989). To be genuine as a leader is to behave without pretense. This means that you are sincere and you do not pretend to be what you are not. You do not hide behind defenses or your leadership role but rather you are authentic and able to honestly share your thoughts and feelings with the group. It is even appropriate at times for the leader to share personal fears or anxieties with the group. This demonstrates to the group that being afraid and anxious is universal and that even you, the leader, experience these feelings. By being genuine yourself you are more likely to elicit the same behavior in others and serve as a role model to encourage genuine behavior in group members (Korda & Pancrazio, 1989). Rogers (1985) cites the following characteristics as being essential to forming a therapeutic relationship: (1) congruence, or genuineness; (2) unconditional positive regard; and (3) accurate empathic understanding. Of these three he believes genuineness to be the most important.

EMPATHY

Although there is one school of thought suggesting that genetic factors may influence a person's ability to be empathic (Matthews, Batson, Horn, & Rosenman, 1981), others believe that the ability to be empathic can be learned and is part of the development of social skills (Yalom, 1983). A person displays empathy when she or he is able to understand and be sensitive to the feelings and experience of others, to "walk in their shoes" and understand their world. When group members experience empathic understanding from the leader or other members, they are more likely to continue sharing and exploring because they feel understood and accepted (Kleinberg, 1991). Goldstein and Myers (1986) view empathic responding as one of the crucial conditions in effecting client change. Supporting this claim are Kassel and Wagner (1993) who, on reviewing literature on self-help groups, found empathy to be one of the major mechanisms to bring about change in members of Alcoholics Anonymous, Parents Anonymous, and Overeaters Anonymous groups. In a survey of occupational therapy educators (Barris &

Kielhofner, 1986), the skill, "be empathic and genuine," was rated the most important of thirty-two skills and techniques judged to be relevant to a psychosocial occupational therapist.

At times it is difficult for a young leader to understand the feelings of a member because she has not yet lived the variety of life situations that come only with age and experience (Posthuma, 1976). However, even young leaders have usually experienced the same emotions, joy, anger, pain, fear, and love even if in other and different situations, so they can still show empathic understanding by being sensitive to and responding to the feelings displayed: "I can see that it is upsetting for you to talk about what happened. It must be very painful." Such a response conveys caring, acceptance, and understanding. Compare it to this response: "I can see that you are upset but you will soon get over it." Responses such as the latter block members from sharing themselves further and prevent them from exploring their experience. Other responses that are nonempathic are critical judgments, blunt questions, telling others how they should or should not feel, being flippant, and/or ignoring a person and moving on to something else.

Two attributes already discussed in this chapter, attending and listening, are central to the empathic process. Sensitive listening, that is demonstrating genuine interest without judgment, is crucial to achieving empathy (Raskin & Rogers, 1989). Empathy can be conveyed nonverbally as well. This can be done with an understanding or caring look, a smile, a touch of the hand, or an arm around the shoulder. Kertay and Reviere (1993) believe that the "use of touch can be, at the very least, a benign form of natural communication . . . and, at best, a means of considerable therapeutic value" (p. 39). Some practitioners feel uncomfortable with touching, often because of being raised in our hands-off society, but if motivated to do so, they can, with practice, become more comfortable as touchers (Posthuma, 1985). While it may be that a person is unable to feel truly empathic with certain individuals, it is important to be compassionate to all. To be compassionate is to respect and care about others, to be sensitive to their feelings and to have a deep concern for their welfare. A compassionate leader offers herself selflessly in the spirit of helping and professionalism.

WARMTH AND CARING

These attributes are noted separately because of their importance even though it is recognized that empathy usually conveys feelings of warmth and caring. Empathy and other helping procedures, however, can be technically correct but when carried out without warmth, they are "therapeutically impotent" (Goldstein & Myers, 1986). Peloquin (1994) says that clients "ask that helpers care, not because concern may cure, but because caring serves humanity" and that "caring attitudes, words, and actions must be at the center of therapeutic practice" (p. 172).

Warmth is an elusive quality to define and yet we all know almost immediately when we encounter a "warm" person. Our senses pick up messages of warmth through various aspects of the person, for example, posture (not rigid), facial expression (smiling), gestures (reaching out for a handshake), tone of voice (modulated), eyes (maintains contact), and mood (receptive). As depicted here, for the most part, warmth is experienced through nonverbal behaviors that tend to stimulate similar responses.

RESPECT

Respect is also an elusive concept to define. Egan (1976) believes it means, "prizing another person simply because he is a human being" (p. 147). Respect is more often displayed through behaviors than through words, as rarely do we actually say "I respect you" to a client or a group member. We can, however, convey this message by showing that we value the member's opinions, ideas, hopes, and feelings. Egan further explains the message of respect as an attitude of being "for" the other person. When group members feel others are for them and are treated courteously and considerately as valued persons, they gain a sense of security and feel freer to participate more fully in the group. It is also the leader's responsibility to see that members show respect for each other. Sometimes this requires intervening to allow a member to finish speaking, interrupting and dealing with any derogatory remarks or behaviors between members (Ferencik, 1992), and monitoring the inclusion of all members.

FLEXIBILITY

If asked, most people would say they are relatively flexible but if they inquire of someone who knows them well, "Do you think I am flexible?," the person is apt to respond, "Well in some things you are, but in others—well . . ." Self-monitoring in this way can be enlightening and constructive and assists you in evaluating your level and areas of flexibility (Ellis & Cronshaw, 1992). By virtue of constantly having to respond to the diverse needs, goals, and limitations of group members a leader must always be in a state of changeableness. Rarely does the process of a group flow smoothly throughout the session or follow precisely a prescribed format. Noncompliance, excitement, dissension, critical incidents, and new and absent members can all challenge the plan and the expectations of the session The leader must be prepared for these exigencies and be able to respond actively and with flexibility. Other instances where a leader may need to call on flexibility could be in:

- Deciding on or changing the task
- Dealing with rules or norms
- Responding to behaviors
- Formalizing structure (i.e., time and place)
- Dealing with other staff
- Coping with peripheral incidents or influences

Collectively the members of a group often form a very diverse assemblage. To be able to interact effectively with so many different personalities requires great flexibility and sensitivity. Diversity may be present in age range as well as in personalities which can precipitate the need for more flexible rules and limits. Indeed, in many facilities the magnitude of the disparity between adolescents and adults is recognized by the establishment of separate units.

The leader should keep an open mind to all ideas, alternatives, and methods and try to avoid the "we've-always-done-it-this-way" manner of thinking. Looking for and responding to new or different ways of "doing" is energizing and stimulates interest and spontaneity.

CREATIVITY AND SPONTANEITY

Closely bound with flexibility is the ability to be creative: to explore new ideas, new methods, and novel approaches. To make the most of such exploring, spontaneity is essential. Just as Moreno (1977) believed that spontaneity was crucial to psychodrama, so is it crucial to the group leader. For example, if the group members reach an impasse in a discussion or interchange, try to problem solve in a creative way. You might think, "Perhaps a role-play could be effective"; act on this idea spontaneously and suggest how the members can get involved. Kottler (1983) notes: "Creative group leaders leave every session bathed in sweat, having squeezed their brains to find new ways of energizing, motivating and facilitating client growth" (p 94).

To be spontaneous does not mean to be impulsive but rather to have the ability to respond assertively in a variety of ways (Egan, 1976). Assertiveness, but not aggression, is essential to spontaneity. In a postgroup discussion of a particular situation the leader will sometimes say, "I thought of trying . . . but . . ." The key is to try it—whatever "it" is, and if it is not effective, feel free to try something else.

ENTHUSIASM

If you are not enthusiastic about the group, group members are not likely to be enthusiastic either. The result? Probably it is a very dull, listless, and boring group. As a role model, show interest in the task or discussion, be energetic, get involved, and encourage members to do the same. This does not mean to take over and "run" the group but rather to be happily and actively *here* as in the "here-and-now." *Enthusiasm* means "to have a zest and excitement for living," or in this context, for the group experience. Many of your group members, by virtue of their illness or life situations, will have lost their zest, drive, and vitality for life. The enthusiasm you display can be contagious, stirring members to engage in more energetic behaviors and interactions. Leaders also are more likely to get personal satisfaction from the group if they embrace their role enthusiastically rather than if they just go through the motions.

HUMOR

Anything that can be done to lighten the load of fellow sufferers is therapeutic (Tooper, 1984). To be able to laugh at one's own predicaments and help others to see the funny side of theirs is an admirable trait. Vergeer and MacRae (1993) found humor to be the "great equalizer" in creating collaborative relationships between clients and practitioners. Through the use of a good-humored manner leaders can show caring while breaking through the barriers presented by some group members. In the same way, they can model more spontaneous behaviors which clients are then able to imitate. It is thought that playfulness and humor can "cut through distance and expand the range of communication, . . . restructure a relationship, or the focus of an interaction" (Ehrenberg, 1991, p. 225).

For many clients life has not been a particularly happy experience. Clients with obsessive, schizoid, or depressive characteristics or those who have been ill for a long time especially tend to be grave and solemn (Bloch, Browning, & McGrath, 1983). Even clients with less onerous problems tend to be earnest and anxious. Because of this many group sessions tend to be serious in tone as members grapple with learning about themselves and their problems. If members can be helped to approach the challenge of changing and learning through a lightening of the mood and by seeing the more humorous aspects of life, then a less arduous process has been facilitated.

The relationship between the painful and the humorous can be viewed as paradoxical in that humor can sometimes be used to alleviate the painful (Tooper, 1984). Among the many messages laughter can convey are warmth, insult, friendliness, bitterness, approval, defiance, exuberance, incredulity, nervousness, shame, embarrassment, and ridicule. According to Kottler (1983), laughter is a means of discharge and as an expressed form of communication has much therapeutic value. Members will sometimes joke and laugh to ease the tension in the group (Orme, 1987) which, depending on the situation, can be either productive or counterproductive. It can be productive if the members are seeking release after an especially intense interchange and the humor serves in a cathartic healing way. Hopefully, there are also times in the group when the members are happy and feeling good and show this by joking, laughing, and just having fun together. However, if the members are joking and laughing to avoid facing up to an intense or important situation, the process can be counterproductive by allowing the members to ignore the issue at hand.

Egan (1976) qualifies the use of humor as a defense by saying it is "probably the least offensive form of resistance" (p. 154). Joking cannot only be used as a way of avoiding the discussion of painful issues, but in some instances can be a means of members bolstering their own self-esteem by putting others down. If this practice is not curtailed, it can turn into scapegoating where one member becomes the butt of all the jokes. Such a situation can be very damaging to the member being picked on and requires the prompt intervention of the leader.

Individuals may also use humour as an avoidance technique. One method of doing this is through self-mockery. However, the member who uses self-mockery as a defense mechanism may find other members joining him in his mockery, causing him to feel inadequate with an even stronger need to defend (Bloch, Browning, & McGrath, 1983). Another way a member may use humor as an avoidance technique is to be the group clown (Burnard, 1992). By constantly joking and clowning around the member is able to keep the other members from taking him or his problems seriously and thus prevents any personal involvement.

At times humor may be introduced through a "fun" task. Banning and Nelson (1987) found that a fun task significantly raised the level of cohesion in groups. In other instances the humorous side of life may only be encountered as the task or discussion unfolds. As long as the leader does not take herself or her role as leader too seriously, she allows herself and enables others to appreciate the human process with all its foibles.

An opposing view of the use of humour comes as a caution to the leader against becoming emotionally involved with a member through a humorous exchange that can dull an objective focus on what is being said. This, of course, can happen among members as well as between a member and the leader. Another problem in using humor, as discussed by Purtilo (1978), is where the leader and a member use humor as a means of gaining control over each other through a game of one-upmanship. What may start out as seemingly harmless banter can only too easily turn into a sarcastic and punitive interaction. The leader must always guard against self-aggrandizement at the expense of the members. Therefore, while the presence of humor is usually welcomed by all concerned, its use should be carefully monitored to ensure that a constructive process is occurring.

CLINICAL REASONING

Although most of the literature and research on clinical reasoning has focused on physicians and a narrow biomedical model of clinical tasks, namely, diagnosis, prognosis, and prescription, the concept is equally relevant to other professionals. Clinical reasoning is an abstract concept which is difficult to describe and impossible to see. *Clinical reasoning* is directed to the human world of motives, values, and beliefs and is referred to as the artful and intuitive process of "putting it all together" (Mattingly, 1991). Thinking about problems and possible solutions presents as a continuous stream of small decisions or temporary hypothesis. Such thinking is often tested in action. For example, if a group member becomes distressed, you may reach out a hand in comfort but should the member withdraw from your touch you are likely to immediately change your approach and perhaps offer verbal support instead. Both these actions have come from your reasoning process.

Fleming (1991) refers to this thinking as the "three-track mind" (Figure 7–1) based on three types of clinical reasoning: (1) procedural, (2) interactive, and (3) conditional. *Procedural* reasoning addresses the known factors about the person's type of illness/problem, how it manifests itself in this person, and what the presenting issues are at this time. *Interactive* reasoning addresses the person as a unique individual and is directed toward understanding the illness or issues from this person's experience and personal point of view (Peloquin, 1993).

Interactive reasoning has been called the "underground practice" and is embodied in the term "therapeutic use of self." It requires analyzing cues from group members, intuitive thinking, and active judgment on several levels simultaneously. It means that the leader must analyze the information she has along with observations of the process occurring in the group to formulate a hypothesis of what is going on. A leader employs *conditional* reasoning to temper or expand her imagining of each member and the group as a whole. The leader imagines how present conditions could change and what members would need to achieve to bring about change, considering strengths and weaknesses along with environmental issues such as the cultural, economic, and family situations of each member and of the members collectively. Reasoning about all these factors constitutes an ongoing process (Schell & Cervero, 1993) within the leader that will affect and be a basis for decisions, actions, and interventions. Engaging a three-track mind leader with a group of 6 members basically requires a person with an 18-track mind—not an easy state to attain!

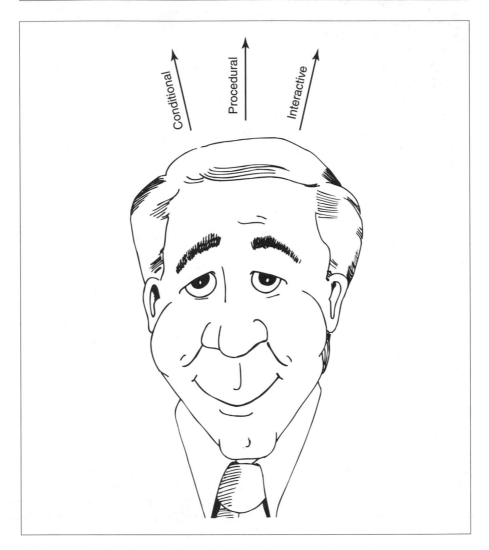

Figure 7–1. The three-track mind of clinical reasoning.

THERAPEUTIC USE OF SELF

As part of clinical reasoning and as more of a personal attribute than a technique, therapeutic use of self is included here. To be *therapeutic* is really to put all the other attributes into action at the most desirable times to meet the needs and facilitate the achievement of the goals of the group members. Urbanowski and Vargo (1994) note that the therapeutic use of self is the primary avenue to connecting with other people's spirituality or their experience of meaning in everyday life. It is a natural use of the self in a manner that empowers both self and others (Fidler, 1993) and in this way will be helpful rather than neutral or harmful.

Another aspect of the therapeutic use of self is the sharing of oneself. This is a controversial issue (McNary & Dies, 1993; Smith, 1990), and must be engaged in sensitively and thoughtfully. By sharing yourself with the group members you become more of a "person" to them which enables them to more easily identify with you (Rachman, 1990). This identification can then lead to members becoming more aware of alternatives, solutions, and coping skills. Conversely, however, because no one is value-free and your sharing is likely to embody your values, it can lead members to feel some pressure to accept or conform to the values you portray. Therefore you must be careful not to lay your values on the members but rather help them explore and clarify their own values (Corey, Corey, & Callanan, 1990a).

Another caution is to share appropriate information or anecdotes at appropriate times. If what you share makes you appear too confident or too competent, then you offer an identity that members will believe to be far out of reach for themselves and so they will feel discouraged rather than encouraged. On the other hand if you frequently disclose fears, problems, and anxieties, you risk presenting an image of a leader who is needy (Frank, 1990), weak, unstable, and perhaps mentally unhealthy (Korda & Pancrazio, 1989). These cautious words are not meant to be inhibiting but hopefully will stimulate a thoughtful awareness as you try to define personal ways of using yourself therapeutically.

SUMMARY

An effective leader can be described as being self-confident, responsible, attentive, objective, genuine, empathic, caring, warm, respectful, flexible, creative, enthusiastic, thoughtful, and as a reasoning person with a sense of humor. These personality dimensions as discussed in this chapter are present to a greater or lesser degree in everyone. While some of these attributes can be seen as inherent personality characteristics, such as self-confidence and a sense of humor, most can be learned or enhanced by direct personal efforts. By keeping these characteristics in mind as you analyze your behavior following each group session, you will gain an awareness of your personal strengths and weaknesses and their effect on your functioning as a leader.

Although "therapeutic use of self" was presented last, it is seen as the most important attribute in becoming an effective leader. It is also the most difficult attribute to define or describe. It is a way of being that mixes and combines sensitivity, intuition, timing, knowing, and courage with all of the other attributes. This combination represents an active and complex process, but ultimately the degree of success achieved in the role of leader will depend on how effectively you are able to integrate all facets of yourself into the situation in a therapeutic manner. Having great self-confidence or a keen sense of humor will be irrelevant if you are unable to use these attributes constructively in concert with your other attributes and the needs of the situation.

Because of the abstractness of the concept it is difficult to delineate what must be learned in order to achieve what is termed the therapeutic use of self. However, from the awareness gained through ongoing self-analysis and self-exploration, you can direct your efforts for personal change toward increasing, improving, and integrating your areas of competency while decreasing any inhibiting attributes. Through this gradual process of change there is likely to evolve a leader who continues to enhance her therapeutic use of self.

Chapter 8

Leadership Techniques

*The real leader . . . is content
to point the way.*
— HENRY MILLER

The attributes discussed in Chapter 7 are primarily personal characteristics, whereas techniques and strategies fall under the term leadership functions. They allow for variety in intervention and constitute skills that can be learned. In describing multimodal therapy Lazarus (1989) suggests that the therapist "uses procedures drawn from different sources without necessarily subscribing to the theories or disciplines that spawned them" (p. 503). This is not to say that the leader should have a bag of tricks from which she pulls out interventions in a hit-or-miss fashion. What it does mean is that the leader will be able to intervene in different ways to assist the members in self-exploration and self-understanding (Corey, 1990). Based on a cognitive-behavioral perspective Conyne, Harvill, Morganett, Morran, and Hulse-Killacky (1990, p. 34) formulated leadership functions which emphasize *thinking* and *doing* while indicating the use of various techniques. These functions are presented here in part:

- Recognition of the need to intervene or not to intervene.
- Generation of plausible alternative interventions.
- Selection of the most appropriate intervention from among the alternatives.
- Communication and application of the intervention in such a manner that it is accurately understood and adequately accepted by the member(s).
- Observation and assessment of group member reactions with appropriate intervention modifications and adjustments.
- Evaluation of the overall intervention effort including self-critique.

In carrying out these functions the leader may use a variety of techniques and strategies depending on the situation in the group at the time. For any leader the most effective techniques will be those that are congruent with her own personal style of leadership and are an extension of the natural "therapeutic use of self." The leader must be sensitive to and able to perceive each group member individually as well as the group as a whole. She must comprehend what is happening and then, when appropriate or necessary, be facilitative by employing the most appropriate technique. The "what is happening" is called the *process,* and as discussed earlier, includes to whom and in what manner members say things, plus all nonverbal behaviors, reactions, and feelings. Following all these occurrences on an ongoing basis is called *processing.* Thus the leader, while being *a part* of the group, must always be *apart* from the group, constantly observing the process. However, it is not enough to only perceive what is occurring in the group; the leader must also help the members acquire some cognitive understanding of the process in order for them to benefit from the experience. The following techniques and strategies, when used by a skilled leader, can facilitate and enhance the group process as well as facilitate members' understanding of the process.

RESTATEMENT

To *restate* what a member has said is basically to repeat a communication using similar language and syntax. The purpose of using this technique is to convey to the member that you are paying close attention and have heard what has been said. It also serves to encourage the member to expand or say more. Example:

STATEMENT: I would like to be more like Bill.

RESTATEMENT: You would like to be more like Bill.

Following the restatement the member may go on to explain how he sees himself and in what ways (personality characteristics or attributes) he would like to be like Bill.

A situation where restating can be particularly useful is if a member is speaking and becomes distracted. When you restate what has just been said, it prods him to continue speaking. It is not a difficult skill to learn but can become sterile and boring if overused.

REFLECTION

Reflecting is the ability to convey the meaning of a member's contribution in such a way as to demonstrate that you both heard and understood. Reflections are not as superficial as restatements. They can focus on the content of what was said or they can reflect the feelings that underlay the communication. Another factor contributing to the complexity of this skill is that it encompasses both verbal and nonverbal messages. Reflecting nonverbal communications can be surprising and enlightening to a member and needs to be done with sensitivity as, used in this way, reflecting can be threatening (Trotzer, 1977). For example, if a member is trying to hide behind a stream of bright chatter but the sadness he really feels is displayed in facial expressions and the latter is reflected by the leader, then the person can feel "found out" and vulnerable. Reflections of lesser impact could be the following:

STATEMENT: I just want to get out of here and go back to work.

REFLECTION: It sounds like you have had enough of this place and would like to get on with your life.

OBSERVATION: Member is shifting in his chair, crossing and uncrossing his legs, swinging his feet.

REFLECTION: It seems like you can't get comfortable; you are fidgeting a lot today.

In reflecting feelings the leader must not appear to be *telling* a member what he is feeling but rather to be *checking* on what the member is feeling. If a member says, "I'm sort of happy, but not really, oh I just don't know" and you respond with, "Sounds like you are feeling a little confused right now" then you leave the communication line open for the member to continue and say more about what he is feeling. If you respond to the above with, "That's OK, we all feel that way sometimes" then you tend to end the communication and the member is less likely to continue. Or, on observing that Mary's eyes are watering and she has stopped talking, the leader might say, "Mary, you look upset." This reflection allows Mary to (1) agree that she is upset, which may lead to a discussion of why she is upset, or (2) deny she is upset, which could lead to exploring just what Mary *is* feeling.

Occasionally a leader can be facilitative by reflecting on the behavior of the group overall, as follows:

LEADER: It seems like everyone is talking at once!

This is an especially useful technique to use if the group members become so caught up in content that they are oblivious of the process. Reflection at this point not only causes a pause in the action of the group but can also be facilitative in producing change.

As with the use of restatement, caution is required to prevent the overuse of reflection which, when carried to its extreme, can become what Corey and Corey (1992) refer to as a "hollow echo." These authors believe that reflection may be a good beginning technique but should be followed by more exploratory interventions. In the following example the first response is a straight reflection, whereas the second includes speculation about causative factors:

STATEMENT: I have to set a date for our wedding pretty soon as Sue won't wait forever.

REFLECTIVE RESPONSE: It sounds like you are afraid Sue might change her mind if you don't agree on a wedding date soon.

EXPLORATORY RESPONSE: It sounds like you are afraid Sue might change her mind but you are still not sure you want to get married.

The exploratory response can be slightly personal and challenging and is more likely to precipitate further dialogue than is the straight reflective response.

PARAPHRASING

Paraphrasing is similar to reflection, which not only makes it easy to confuse the two but hampers clearly differentiating between them. *Paraphrasing* addresses the major communication problem that occurs when people assume that what they understood another person to say is actually what the other person intended to say. In responding to others most people speak from their own understanding of what the other person meant without checking to see if they *heard* the message or the intention correctly. On hearing a new telephone number, we often repeat it to check for accuracy, but with other communications we usually assume that we heard correctly what was said.

To make sure that the meaning you take from another person's remark is the meaning intended, you can check by asking, "Can you clarify that?" or, "Is this (statement) what you meant?" You can also paraphrase what was said to show the other person what the statement meant to you; for example:

MEMBER: My husband is very nasty to me.

LEADER: He physically abuses you?

MEMBER: No, he doesn't do that, but he constantly laughs and sneers at me.

This paraphrase by the leader leads to a clarification of what the member meant by "nasty." However, if the leader had said, "He is mean to you?" the member might have said "Yes." The leader would still not know specifically what the husband does when he is being nasty and may assume that he physically abuses the member. So, when paraphrasing, it is very important to be specific, to try to state exactly what the other person is saying.

Another reason paraphrasing is a useful tool in communication is that it conveys interest in the other person. It is evidence that you want to understand what the other person is saying. Because paraphrasing does convey a message of interest the other person may be more inclined to open up and share. Paraphrasing comes from a genuine desire to understand what another person means and is one of the best ways to increase accuracy in communication.

CLARIFYING

The responsibility of clarifying what an individual member says or what the group is doing often falls to the leader. You can be sure that if you do not understand something that has been said or done there will be others who do not understand. They, however, may not feel comfortable saying so. In such instances it is important to facilitate understanding by *clarifying*. When Joe says, "I don't want to be in group," it is not clear whether he is uncomfortable with this particular session, has something pressing he wants to do right now, or just generally dislikes being part of the group. If let pass, such an ambiguous statement by Joe can affect how the other members relate to him. To clarify you might ask, "Joe, do you mean just today?" Hopefully, his answer will clear up the confusion surrounding his previous statement, enabling everyone to feel more comfortable with Joe and the situation.

Sometimes clarifying the overall process in the group is required. If the members seem to be going in different directions with the discussion or task, the question, "Can someone explain what we are doing right now?" may precipitate clarification and render a clearer focus. Other clarifiers might be: "Is the problem deciding who will do what?" or "Have we decided on how to begin?" Intervening in these or similar ways can be facilitative in helping members define immediate goals and decide how to proceed. There are times when members will get caught up in a game of semantics and then a clarifying statement can often end the confusion. Paraphrasing and restatement, as discussed previously, also can be effective methods of clarifying.

SUPPORT

Offering *support* is a means of encouraging an individual member or the group as a whole. Support should be proffered in both good times and bad times—that is, when the group (or a member) is thought to be doing well, and when they (or a member) appear to be in difficulty. There will be times when a person, finding it painful to explore an issue or deal with a situation, appears to stop or pull back. This could be an instance where offering some support might be appropriate and appreciated. To be supportive the leader might say something like, "It's difficult to deal with such a tough issue by yourself. Maybe we can help." To the group, the leader might offer encouragement (e.g., "As a group you are working very hard and I'm sure it's not easy."). Supportive statements let the group (member) know that: (1) you are listening, (2) what they are saying is valued, and (3) you are aware of their feelings. Sometimes this is all that is necessary for the group or member to feel able to carry on. Feeling confident that what they say will be recognized and responded to they feel more comfortable in continuing or initiating.

Creating a supportive climate in the group is important in enabling the members to feel comfortable in sharing their ideas and feelings and in exploring new avenues. It is more likely that members will share what they deem to be the unacceptable parts of themselves or their lives in a supportive environment (Jacobs, Harvill, & Masson, 1988). By offering supportive comments at appropriate times, the leader serves as a role model, and group members may then follow suit by being supportive of their peers. However, giving support at inappropriate times, such as when a member is looking for unwarranted sympathy or is being overly dependent, can be counterproductive. The skill then is not only in being able to be supportive but in knowing when such an intervention will be constructive.

TIMING

We have all heard it said that a certain person's "timing was right" and that is why Tim was successful or why things went so well for him. Similarly, in a group, for things to go well, the timing of interventions is a crucial factor. Although *timing* is one of the most important skills for a leader to develop (Hansen, Warner, & Smith, 1980), there are no rules to follow or guidelines to go by. Skill in this technique comes with practice and experience. The following points may serve as useful guidelines. As with all leadership techniques, timing must be based on the process occurring in the group at the time—any intervention must be congruent with what is going on in the group at that particular moment. More to the point, the intervention must be congruent with the personal state of any specific individual who is directly involved. For example, if a member is being very defensive and the leader pushes an issue, the intervention may only serve to make the member more defensive. So, not only must the intervention be congruent but it should be made at the *optimal* time. To intervene too early in a discussion can cut off or stifle the interaction, but to wait too long is to risk losing the facilitative aspect of the intervention. For instance, if feelings are building among members in the group and the leader intervenes too early, then the members can opt out by entering into interaction with the leader rather than continuing the discussion with one another. This allows their feelings to dissipate and resolution can be lost. At other times, however, it will be more productive for the leader to make the intervention early in order to prevent feelings from escalating. The skill is to recognize the differences in the two situations and to intervene accordingly.

In considering another kind of group where the discussion is more one of brainstorming or idea exchange, the leader faces the same question of when (if at all) to intervene. In this case you might look for more objective criteria:

- Are group members getting too far off the topic?
- Is the interaction among the members more important (for the moment) than staying on the topic?
- Are most members or only a few involved in the exchange?

Weighing these or other factors will help the leader decide when and how to intervene. Often you will be able to tell from the reaction of the group members whether your timing was facilitative or not. If members ignore your input, you can pretty much conclude that your timing was off. Conversely, if the group responds by incorporating your input and carrying on, then you have probably been on target.

It is said elsewhere in this book but is worth repeating: as a rule of thumb, it is better to err on the side of too few interventions than too many. New leaders often tend to be too active because they feel responsible for keeping the group going and attempt to do so by intervening or contributing in some manner. A situation that tends to precipitate poorly timed interventions by a novice leader is when there is protracted silence in the group. Because of the degree of their discomfort, new leaders frequently have a distorted sense of the duration of the silence and believe it to be much longer than it is in fact.

A last important point about timing is *time* itself. The leader needs to keep an eye on the clock to ensure sufficient time is left to allow for a smooth approach to closure. If the members are into a heavy discussion and group time is almost up, it is important to intervene in an effort to help members resolve the issue and deal with their individual feelings within the remaining time. In some facilities, due to staff or program requirements, groups must stop exactly on time. If members are left feeling up in the air because of unfinished business, this can be unproductive, both for them individually and for the milieu of the group.

Sometimes, but again not always, it is helpful to let the group know how much time remains and to indicate the need to finish up—"There are five minutes left so we need to think about closing" or "We have ten minutes left to share our thoughts and feelings on this." The value of such interventions depends on what is going on in the group at the time and the manner in which the intervention is made. In certain instances such an intervention can inhibit members' participation and the group may come to an abrupt end. At other times it may facilitate members to get to the point, make decisions, or move to supportive and summary comments, bringing the group to a comfortable and productive close.

QUESTIONS, STATEMENTS, AND PROBING

Many of the personal qualities and therapeutic skills that produce a successful interview are the same as those required to effect a productive group session. However, because of this similarity and because counselors and therapists are used to interviewing, it is easy for the leader to fall into an interview format with individual members of the group. A barrage of cognitive questions cannot only alter the tone of a group by preventing the expression of feelings (Clark, 1989) but can also encourage members to become leader dependent.

The directing as well as the phrasing of questions has important implications. Asking questions of a specific member of the group may invite a one-to-one interaction with the member. Of course this cannot always be avoided nor need it be. There are times when issues need to be explored with certain members or specific individuals need to be drawn out. Points to ponder at these times are the duration of the dialogue, whether the rest of the group is excluded, and if the content of the discussion can be broadened to include some of the other members.

Burnard (1992) defines two main types of questions: open and closed. The question, "How would the group like to handle it?" is considered open and more facilitative than, "Would you like to go around the circle taking turns?"—a closed question. You may get a variety of responses and ideas to the first question, but probably only a yes or no from the second. The second question keeps you in the position of control whereas the first gives control to the group and lets them decide what to do. A third type, a directive question, requests information about ideas being discussed; for example, "What are the advantages of the group meeting in the afternoon?" Directive questions are useful in encouraging members to explore alternatives and assess options. As in any interactive situation, the following types of questions should be avoided whenever possible: "why" questions, leading questions, and value-laden questions (Burnard, 1992).

Statements also can be productive. The statement, "I think we could explore this further," is more likely to produce more discussion than, "Do you think we have covered the issue?" The latter has more of a closing-off tone, whereas the first denotes a sense of opening up. This is not to say there are not times when you do want to close off the discussion and therefore would deliberately choose to use the question rather than the statement. Shoemaker's (1987) research demonstrates that by "varying the focus of interventions and the pattern of communication" (p. 36), the leader can significantly affect the type of learning that occurs. Keeping inquiries varied and fresh will contribute to input and interaction being more stimulating and provocative.

Questioning can also be a form of avoidance behavior (Sklare, Keener, & Mas, 1990) when used defensively by group members. Members may avoid sharing information about themselves by asking for information from others. Initially such questioning may appear positive as it appears to indicate interest and does create interactions among members. As the process continues and the defensive pattern emerges, however, it is best to intervene. Leaders can help members convert questions to statements by encouraging them to explore what they themselves feel about the issue/situation. At first members may feel taken aback by the leader's suggestion but in time they seem to realize that statements elicit more direct communication.

Aside from the risks, questioning and probing can enable group members to explore and expand their awareness in order to reach deeper levels of understanding. They are useful in encouraging members to generate new ideas and alternatives, to aid in developing the topic, and to promote deeper levels of relating. Probing can take the form of direct questions, statements, or phrases:

- How did that make you feel?
- That sounds stressful.
- And then?

As with the other techniques, the leader must use probing with a good deal of sensitivity. It can be very threatening to group members and if done too directly or forcefully, members can feel pushed or picked on, and they may withdraw or respond defensively.

CONTENT VERSUS PROCESS

As mentioned previously, it is crucial that the leader be constantly aware of the dynamics unfolding in the group. Included should be an awareness of how you are affecting the group and how you are being affected by the group. Concurrent to being *aware* of the process you must *monitor* the process, be it a discussion or an active task. Sometimes, a member will bring up an issue or topic having great personal relevance and interest to you. In such instances there can be a natural tendency to get completely caught up in the discussion, to forget your leadership role as you become totally involved with the content. This can present a problem in that it leaves no one to "mind the store," and as *you* become more active, other group members may pull back. At this point you may find yourself in the position of "lecturing" to the group on your favorite topic, or sliding into an exclusive one-to-one discussion with a particular member. So, while it is important to pay attention and be involved in the content, it is equally important to remain observant and objective.

BITING YOUR TONGUE

Throughout the course of any one group session the leader will hear information and observe behaviors that immediately stimulate a desire to respond or comment. To constantly react to these feelings will make you a very active leader. Frequently it will be more conducive to the development of the group if you bide your time. However, because most counselors and therapists are caring individuals, it can be difficult as a leader to watch your group flounder and not jump in to bail them out. Difficult as it may be, biting your tongue is often the most productive course to take. It is stressful to do this because as practitioners we are used to solving problems, directing treatment, and generally participating actively with our clients. On average, in a group setting, it is often more productive for your members, both individually and as a group, to work things out and solve their own problems. It may take them longer, doing it themselves, but their gains in learning and the added feelings of competency are very rewarding.

The benefits of pulling back will vary with the different stages of the group. In a first session or even at the beginning of each new session it is likely that you will need to be fairly active to help members mobilize themselves. Once members begin to feel somewhat comfortable with the setting and with each other, decreasing your activity level will enable the group to assume more responsibility. A good rule of thumb is to "wait and see" for a minute or two before jumping in or rescuing—they may be able to do it themselves.

FEEDBACK

The well-known lines of Robert Burns, "O wad some power the giftie gie us, to see oursel's as ithers see us," intimate our hunger to know how others perceive us. People want to know how they are seen by others in order to validate or, at times, invalidate their self-perceptions (Kenny & De Paulo, 1993). Group members have the opportunity to meet these needs when a feedback process is activated in the group. They can determine the effects of their behaviors and ways of interrelating with others from the feedback they receive. Having more than one's own point of view can be seen as advantageous in the cognitive structuring or restructuring of a person's behavior. To consolidate this new learning, Edelwich and Brodsky (1992, p. 141) suggest that the group leader ask the following three questions:

1. What did you hear each person say?
2. What have you learned from this feedback?
3. What are you going to do about it?

Although it is generally assumed that most people welcome feedback it should be kept in mind that people do differ in the *degree* of their desire for feedback (Snyder, Ingram, Handelsman, & Wells, 1982). This means that some group members will be more receptive to receiving feedback than will others and it is important, as leader, to be prepared for varied reactions. People also tend to accept positive feedback and believe in its accuracy more readily than they do negative feedback (Handelsman & Snyder, 1982); the latter, therefore, is more likely to precipitate defensive behavior. Giving feedback is a skill requiring sensitivity. By keeping the following points in mind a leader can facilitate a more meaningful and effective feedback process.

1. *Be sensitive* to what information the group is ready to use. Give feedback that will be most helpful *to the group* at the time. The behaviors and incidents observed as most significant by *you* will not necessarily be the ones the group is ready to hear about.

2. *Do not "avalanche"* the group with information. If too much information is given at one time, the group will find it overwhelming and barely useful. Because of their confusion the members may even ignore all the feedback.

3. *Do not overpraise* the group. Be selective and give praise on specifics; otherwise members may feel they have "made it" and therefore need make no further efforts.

4. *Try not to punish, preach, or judge.* Instead of saying, "Some of you dominated the discussion today," say, "It was interesting that participation was less general today than it was last session."

5. *Feedback should be immediate.* Give feedback when the behavior occurs rather than waiting until the end of the group to comment. Saying: "That was a very helpful suggestion Mary," "I find it very distracting when you keep tapping your fingers," or "You are very quiet today" allows the member in question an opportunity to repeat or change behavior during the remainder of the group.

6. *Use confrontive feedback carefully* in the beginning of a group. Early confrontation can frighten members and inhibit them from further participation. This is not to say that disruptive behaviors should be overlooked during this time. They should be confronted immediately or as warranted.

7. *Act as a role model* for giving feedback like the following:

LEADER (TO JOHN): I'm finding it difficult to concentrate when you keep tapping your fingers. *(To group)* "Is it bothering anyone else?"

MEMBER: Yes

LEADER: Could you tell John that?

By speaking to John yourself initially you demonstrate that it is acceptable to give this sort of feedback and members will then feel more comfortable in following your lead.

Feedback can be given to the group as a whole as well as to individuals. It helps to keep the group focused (e.g., "We seem to be getting off topic"), balances affect with content ("You seem to be avoiding saying how you feel about these issues"), and clarifies process ("I notice that John always speaks for the group"). It has been shown that congruency between the type of goals (individual or group) and type of feedback (individual or group) can affect the group's performance (Saavedra, Earley, & Van Dyne, 1993). To give feedback on individual performance during a group task can be damaging not only to the person being picked on but to the overall interdependence of the group members. In all cases feedback should be descriptive rather than evaluative or judgmental. In addition, it is most useful when it has a here-and-now rather than a there-and-then focus. It is more difficult to deny or argue with behaviors that can be pinpointed and described as they occur. Once their existence has been established, then their effect on then-and-there situations can be hypothesized and discussed.

It is also important for leaders to listen for and accept feedback from group members (Nelson-Jones, 1990b). In this way leaders can gain valuable information on how to change, modify, and improve their style and methods of leadership. To become defensive in the face of feedback from group members defeats your effectiveness as a role model and interferes with your own learning.

CONFRONTATION

Confrontation is also a form of feedback. Whether a member says a benign, "You are speaking too softly," or a much stronger, "You interrupted me," the member is functioning in a confrontational role. *Confrontation* is a means of prompting individuals to examine their behaviors, of breaking through defenses, and of increasing awareness. It is a skill requiring practice to ensure that its use will be facilitative and not destructive. Unfortunately, the word confrontation has a rather negative connotation, but the actual act of confronting need not produce a negative experience for those involved. In confronting a member or the group you can be straightforward and direct, but you need not be abrasive. One of the main things to be aware of in confronting another person is your tone of voice. An even, low voice will help to present your confrontation in a sensitive and caring way. Kreps and Thornton (1984) offer four components of constructive confrontation: (1) clarifying the issue, (2) expressing feelings descriptively, (3) expressing facts and fantasies, and (4) resolution and agreement (p. 186). These are in keeping with the previous suggestions for offering constructive feedback.

The leader can use confrontation as a means of letting an individual or the whole group know that she is aware of what is going on. In this way the leader can make the point while simultaneously serving as a role model in demonstrating confrontive behaviours for the group members (Burnard, 1992). For example, in a certain group a member called Tony is always blaming others or poor circumstances for his problems and what he sees as his misfortunes. The leader believes that the other members are aware of Tony's behavior but are reluctant to confront him. The following illustrates how the leader might deal with the situation:

TONY: I didn't get the job because the fellow who interviewed me didn't ask the right questions and he ended the interview too soon.

LEADER: Tony, I feel we've heard this sort of reasoning from you before. I'm wondering if you are aware that when things go wrong for you, you often seem to think it is someone else's fault.

TONY: Well it was. If he'd asked the right questions and given me more time, I could have got the job.

LEADER: Tony, you are still blaming someone else and this seems to be the way you often react to avoid accepting responsibility for your own behavior. Let's hear what the others think about what you've said.

With the leader's second response she is making an interpretation of Tony's behavior as a means of emphasizing the point to be made. In doing this she may initiate an involved one-to-one interaction with Tony that could exclude the rest of the group. By referring the issue to the group, as she does at the end of her second response, the leader will hopefully extricate herself from the dialogue while stimulating the group members to follow on with their feedback to Tony. This can strengthen the message to be conveyed.

Most important, any confrontation should "manifest your concern for the other" (Egan, 1983). Used punitively or insensitively it is sure to cause the individual or the group to retreat. Confrontation should always convey caring and function as a means of increasing involvement.

ANALYSIS AND INTERPRETATION

Observation is the forerunner to analysis, and analysis is the forerunner to interpretation. It is important to separate observations from interpretations. The leader must be able to differentiate what she sees and hears from what she thinks these observations mean (Sampson & Marthas, 1981). You should not be hasty in making interpretations but should *analyze* personal observations over time and under various circumstances. For example, if John is smiling, you might infer that he is happy, but on further observation you find that John also smiles when he is being confronted or is relating a sad experience. On analyzing several of these situations you might then conclude that John uses smiling as a defense mechanism. Interpreted, this could mean that John is unable or unwilling to experience or express his real feelings. Continued interaction with John may supply more clues and information on which to base further interpretations.

It is important to present any interpretation as a hunch or a hypothesis rather than as a statement of fact. Therefore interpretations are often prefaced with the words "it seems" or "it appears." This way the validity of the interpretation is open to agreement or disagreement, acceptance or rejection by the member involved. An interpretation, if accurate, can be useful in moving a member or the group past an impasse as it opens up a new way of looking at or evaluating the situation or issue (Corey & Corey, 1992).

Interpretation is frequently used to help persons gain insight into why they behave the way they do. It is most often used in the psychoanalytic approach to psychotherapy but is a useful technique for any leader. To make an inaccurate interpretation is not a calamity. The member or group will usually set you straight about the error and then together you can explore other possibilities. Even when your interpretation is judged to be off base, there is the possibility that it contains a grain of truth that could give the member or group some food for thought. The leader need not always be the one to make an interpretation. In some cases it may be more beneficial for the member to attempt to interpret his own behavior. The leader might encourage the member to do so by saying, "John, what do you think is the reason that you always make a joke when Bill talks about his mother?"

In analyzing what is going on in the group or with individuals, many aspects must be considered: the order and context of events, interrelationships, nonverbal behaviors, verbal behaviors, actions, and affect. Good observational skills, steady concentration, and acute awareness are all necessary in order to absorb and analyze the total dynamics of the group. Sometimes presenting the analysis to the group will motivate the members themselves to examine what is going on in the group. For example, you notice that whenever a member gives what could be construed as some negative feedback to another member, the rest of the group jumps in immediately with positive feedback for the member. By making this observation you are presenting the group with an analysis of what you perceive to be happening in the group. You are not saying *why* it is happening, but only that it *is* happening. Such an analysis can be effective in breaking up the pattern of behaviors occurring in the group and moving the members on to more productive behaviors. Chapter 12 discusses group analysis more fully.

SUMMARIZING FOR THE GROUP

Although we usually associate a summary with completion, it can be useful to summarize at various points during a group. At the beginning of the session you may choose to briefly summarize what happened during the previous session and what learnings occurred (Nelson-Jones, 1992). During the session if the group has exhausted a topic or is floundering, summarizing what has been discussed can help the members decide if there is more to be said or if it is time to move on. To summarize the points made by various group members can be especially facilitative if the group is involved in a decision making process or in a task requiring several steps. The summary can prod the group to complete one step or begin the next one.

Near the close of a session you might make a summary statement about how you thought the group went, and check if your perceptions match those of the members. Other ways of closing could be to ask if someone in the group would like to summarize the session, or alternatively to discuss how you yourself are feeling at the close of the session and invite others to do the same. This latter method helps assess how members are feeling before they leave the group and serves as a check for unfinished business or unresolved feelings.

SUMMARY

A leader will be most effective if she can remain objective and guard against getting personally caught up in either the content or the process. This can be done by monitoring both areas separately and continually, and then when appropriate, responding to the needs of each with facilitative techniques. This is not to say that the leader should not offer herself personally or should refrain from contributing. However, it does mean that entering into an argument with a member or telling the group what the right answer or right way is can, in the former instance, be a destructive maneuver and in the latter, be inhibiting to the sharing of ideas. Becoming personally involved also takes the leader out of the role of observer and places her in the role of *powerful member*—powerful because of the given role of leader. This latter role carries great influence as well as the concept of knowing and therefore the leader is often perceived by members to be an "expert." Usually it is more productive to observe and to facilitate the process among members than to intervene as an expert and risk terminating it. Members may take time to get it right, but they are more likely to retain any learning that occurs if they go through the process themselves.

In addition to the personal characteristics, as discussed in Chapter 7, that are conducive to effective leadership, there are techniques and strategies that can be learned and used as ongoing methods or at appropriate junctures during a group session. The techniques presented here facilitate interaction processes and outcomes. Some, such as supporting, clarifying, questioning, and biting your tongue, will be more familiar and hence more comfortable to use than others. As a rule, normal, accepted social skills do not include confronting, probing, giving feedback, or analyzing or interpreting the behavior of others and so these techniques, besides requiring theoretical knowledge, may require conscious practice. Still other techniques, specifically restatement, reflection, and paraphrasing, contribute to more effective communication and increased understanding between participators and skill with the use of these techniques can enhance any relationship.

Chapter 9

Theoretical Approaches

*No theory is good except on condition
that one use it to go on beyond.*
— ANDRE GIDE

Each would-be group leader must explore and develop a theoretical perspective on which to base a personal leadership style (Corey, 1990). Most group leaders will develop personal styles and techniques of leading based on their knowledge, skills, and comfort levels. These styles will differ from leader to leader based on individual preferences, experience, and ability. This perspective need not, and one might say should not (De Pree, 1987), be based on one theory alone but does require an understanding and grasp of concepts germane to the various theories that one is drawing on. Certain theoretical approaches will appeal more to some than to others. These preferences are often formed through the assimilation of socially popular beliefs, educators' biases, and personal experience.

Most theoretical models of group work are based on theories of psychotherapy that were developed and used initially for individual psychotherapy. These same theories, however, are considered to be applicable and adaptable to group work (Vacc, 1989). It should be mentioned though, that one of the hazards of extending the theory into a group setting is that individual therapy may continue between the leader and members of the group in turn. To do this negates the purpose and value of group process and the group setting and will greatly limit the effectiveness of any session. To be effective, techniques and procedures of the various psychotherapeutic approaches must be extended, transported, and adapted into group concepts.

There are many theories from which a beginning leader may draw and extended exploration of the literature is encouraged. However, only four of these approaches are reviewed here and then only briefly as it is anticipated that the reader will be somewhat familiar with this information or can access it from other sources (Corey, 1990; Corsini & Wedding, 1989). The theoretical models selected were chosen for their differences and for their

Table 9–1. Comparative Group Approaches

Approach	Leader Behavior	Therapeutic Focus	Leader–Member Relationship	Contents
Client-centered	Nondirective, conveying warmth, empathy, acceptance, active listening, paraphrasing, linking	Subjective experiences; somewhat intrapsychic	Warm, open, positive, friendly, companionable	Anxieties, feelings, relationships, personal experiences
Behavioral	Reinforcing, modeling, limit setting	Specific behaviors	Contracting, businesslike, straightforward	Symptoms, anxieties, problems, overt behaviors, rehearsal for new behaviors
Psychoanalytic	Nondirective, passive interpreting, probing	Intrapsychic events	Vague, changeable, spontaneous, health professional–client	Symptoms, life events, free association
Rational–emotive	Active, directive, confronting, persuading, challenging	Irrational thoughts, values, beliefs	Tolerant, impersonal, teacher–learner	Cognitions, behaviors, attitudes, belief systems

Source: Adapted from J. L. Shapiro, *Methods of group psychotherapy: A tradition of innovation*. Itasca, IL: F. E. Peacock, 1978.

importance and relevance to effective group leadership. Table 9–1 presents a concise comparative overview of these selected theoretical approaches.

PERSON-CENTERED THERAPY

Person-centered therapy was developed from the theories of self-actualization that re-emerged in the mid-twentieth century, and stems primarily from the work of Carl Rogers (Corey, 1990). Originally known as client-centered or nondirective therapy, the client or person is the central figure in this form of therapy. The key factor is the belief that the individual can be trusted to take responsibility for his or her own life without the direct intervention of a therapist (Ginsberg, 1984). Rogers emphasized the need for an open, honest, caring, accepting, and nonjudgmental attitude on the part of the therapist. He believed that the key to a successful therapeutic outcome was the quality of the client–therapist relationship (Rogers, 1961). In groups he conceptualized the leader's role "as exemplifying the same basic qualities as the individual therapist; in addition he thought it important to accept and respect the group as a whole" (Raskin & Rogers, 1989; p. 182). He maintained that the three conditions necessary for a growth-promoting therapeutic climate were (1) genuineness and realness, (2) unconditional positive regard, and (3) empathy or understanding (Rogers, 1985).

Leader Functions/Techniques

Because of its nondirective aspects the group-centered approach allows the leader to do less "leading" with the result being increased participation by the group members. Rogers (1951) describes five distinctive functions carried out by the group-centered leader: (1) conveying warmth and empathy, (2) attending to others, (3) understanding meanings and intents, (4) conveying acceptance, and (5) linking.

Conveying Warmth and Empathy   It is difficult to describe just how a leader behaves to convey warmth and empathy but it appears to be behaviors and attitudes that manifest themselves in the leader's facial expressions, gestures, and speech. This basic manner in how the leader comes across is of utmost importance in creating a nonthreatening, accepting atmosphere. Rogers (1985) believed that the overall emotional tone of any group could be greatly affected by the degree of warmth and empathy displayed by the leader. When group members identify with the leader, they often internalize the same attitudes and behaviors the leader displays. This means that group members will gradually become friendlier, warmer, and more empathic in their interactions with one another. Such conditions greatly enhance the quality and degree of communication in a group.

Attending to Others   Most group members do not naturally possess effective listening skills. They find the act of listening attentively to another person a difficult task. This lack of skill emanates from a life's experience of focusing and working hard on our verbal expressions while, for the most part,
ignoring our receptive abilities (Barrett-Lennard, 1988). Instead of attending,
members are thinking ahead and formulating their responses or additional
input. It is a common occurrence in groups for several members to succes-
sively bring up different points or ideas, none of which relate to the others.
In such instances it is clear that the members are not attending to what others are saying. This lack of attention from others can cause some members
to withdraw and refrain from participating because they sense their contributions are not being heard or welcomed (Natiello, 1987).

The group-centered leader, by virtue of not needing to present or force
personal views, is free to listen attentively to the contributions of each group
member. The possession of the ability to closely attend to members is considered a primary skill of the group-centered leader. Trotzer (1977) expands
this consideration by believing active listening to be the primary reaction skill
for *all* group leaders and believes this is the behavior that conveys acceptance, respect, caring, and empathic understanding to the group members.
These messages will not be conveyed if the leader is thinking:

- Are the members doing what I want them to do?
- I don't think what he said is true.
- I wonder if they like me?
- How can I get Mary involved?
- That is not important.

Given that active listening is a crucial interactive skill, then the question
becomes, "How do you convey the message that you are really attending to
what another is saying?" Such cues as looking directly at the person, nodding
the head, and offering some "uh-huh's" are helpful, but one can do these and
still not be listening. As an aside, one can also respond with "yes" or "uh-
huh" and be misunderstood. Foy (1994) points out the difference that gender can make in the interpretation of such responses. She says that during a
conversation between a man and a woman in a business or social context
when a woman says "yes" (meaning that she understands), the man hears "I
agree." Many other discrepancies that occur during conversations between
men and woman are described by D. Tannen (1990) and have relevance for
interactions among group members and between members and the leader.

Then there are the people who are very good at appearing attentive
while their thoughts are miles away. However, if the listener reflects what
has been said, then the speaker knows that she or he has been listened to.
On receiving such undivided attention the member feels respected because
Tom feels his contribution was received and is worthwhile. Leaders using

a group-centered approach frequently begin their responses with phrases similar to:

> You are saying . . .
>
> You feel . . .
>
> If I understand you correctly . . .
>
> I gather that you mean . . .
>
> I'm not sure I follow you, but is it that . . .
>
> Let's see if I really understand that . . .

Gradually group members pick up this ability to attend by checking for understanding and meaning in what has been said by others. It can be very helpful in promoting interaction when members assume some of the responsibility for listening to others in this way. In terms of process, this involvement of the members is important as it allows the leader to relinquish parts of the leadership role and avoid the development of one-to-one dialogues with members. Passing on the skills of attending and reflecting to the members is thought to be a distinctive contribution, unique to group-centered leaders.

Understanding Meanings and Intents As important as listening and reflecting are, these skills are not enough if people do not say what they mean, as is often the case. The leader then must try to bring out the "secret intent" of what has been said. By paraphrasing what the member has said, the leader may help the member realize what is "really meant."

JOE: I think we should end group early today. I'm tired.

LEADER: You're feeling too tired to stay with us any longer.

JOE: Well, I don't know if I'm tired or bored.

LEADER: You don't know if you're really tired or just tired of what's going on.

JOE: Yeah, we haven't been talking about anything important.

LEADER: So, the last little while has been pretty uninteresting for you.

JOE: Yeah, it was better in the last group when we talked about things that make us angry.

LEADER: You found that discussion more helpful. Let's see how the others feel about that.

From this exchange it appears that Joe did not really want to leave the group but rather wanted to talk about something else—perhaps more about anger. Joe may not have realized this initially and thus could not say this outright. He was only aware of the fact that he did not like what was going on. The leader, through paraphrasing, enabled Joe to grapple with and then finally identify what actually promoted his statement. If the leader, in response to Joe's first statement, "I think we should end the group early today. I'm tired," had said something like, "It's only fifteen more minutes, I think you should try and stay," then Joe is cut off. As a result, he may feel reprimanded and withdraw even further. When the leader uses paraphrasing to help Joe clarify his feelings, Joe feels accepted and encouraged to continue. Joe is finally able to express the real meaning and intent behind his desire to end the group.

Conveying Acceptance   In person-centered therapy, the therapist conveys complete acceptance of the person, and so must the group-centered leader convey acceptance of the individual members and the group. The leader must accept the group as it is at the moment and "convey a genuine acceptance of what the group members wish to discuss, what they decide to do and how they plan to do it" (Rogers, 1951, p. 355). This is not to say that the leader must be accepting if the members behave in ways that are malevolent or destructive and therefore totally unacceptable to the leader. In fact the group-centered leader is accepting "within limits" and these limits will depend on the boundaries of human decency, the structure and standards of the facility, and the values of the leader. However, because of the group-centered leader's belief in the abilities of the group members, she sets fewer limits than a leader who believes that the group needs to be tightly controlled. Group members who experience acceptance from the leader are likely to become more accepting and tolerant of their fellow group members. This accepting environment creates trust among members and promotes the sharing and exchange of genuine thoughts and sincere feelings in the group.

Linking   The act of connecting the meaning of what one group member says to the meaning of what another member says is called *linking*. This skill depends largely on the insightfulness of the leader in ferreting out common themes or feelings from what different members say (Nelson-Jones, 1992). To describe linking, Rogers (1951) uses the analogy of raindrops falling on a windowpane. Each raindrop represents a contribution by a group member and just as a raindrop forms a course of its own down the windowpane, so may each member's input stand alone. However, by using one's finger one can link up one raindrop's flow with that of another one, creating an enlarged raindrop that may or may not find a new course. The interaction-oriented leader can, in a similar fashion, link the thoughts of one member to those of another and as this process flourishes, the discussion gains strength and meaning as new contributions are linked in. For example, if Mary is sharing the despair she feels since her husband left her, the group-oriented leader could comment that her sense of loss and abandonment might be similar to the feelings experienced by Jim when his boss fired him or the way Anne felt when her parents asked her to move out. Linking in this way can facilitate interaction, sharing, and understanding among group members which in turn can raise the level of group cohesion (Corey & Corey, 1992). Sometimes the commonality of contributions is hidden and the leader, by clarifying the meaning of a comment, can facilitate the linking of ideas and promote a more encompassing discussion.

BEHAVIOR THERAPY

Within the behavioral perspective there are a variety of procedures but the basic assumption of this approach is that "all problematic behaviors, cognitions, and emotions have been learned and that they can be modified by new learning" (Corey, 1990, p. 383). The basic constructs of reinforcement and extinction are among those most widely understood and universally applied (Waldinger, 1990). When working individually with clients, counselors and therapists frequently employ tactics based on these two constructs. Practitioners who praise a client's particular behavior—"It's nice to see you smiling this morning, Bob"—know the value of reinforcement in encouraging a client to continue or repeat his effort. They also know that if they consistently ignore undesirable behavior, there is a good possibility that the behavior will eventually disappear.

These two constructs of behavior therapy, when employed in a small group setting, can be equally if not more effective than when used individually. In a group there is the opportunity for reinforcement to come not only from the leader but from the other group members as well. Such "multiple" reinforcement naturally carries a stronger message and therefore increases the impact of the message and the likelihood that change will occur. The same holds true for attempts at eliminating unacceptable behaviors. If the leader ignores a certain behavior exhibited by a member, the other group members are likely to follow this example and ignore the member's behavior as well. The individual, feeling ignored by both members and the leader, may abandon his unacceptable behavior to regain a sense of acceptance.

Leader Functions/Techniques

Methods of behavior therapy that are particularly effective in advancing therapeutic outcomes in a group are contracting, cognitive restructuring, and modeling.

Contracting   Contracting, or drawing up an agreement with another person, can be an effective way to help clients who are having problems with some or all parts of the group experience. For example, an apathetic client may be experiencing difficulties such as getting to group on time, speaking in group, or staying for the specified period of time. If the member's lateness is especially disruptive, the leader may initiate the formulation of a contract between the member and the group. Following a discussion of the problem, including how tardiness affects the leader, other group members, and even the individual, an oral (or written) contract is suggested.

The contract, which contains behavioral objectives dealing with punctuality, will be an agreement between the tardy member and the total group. Through this contract, the member is actually saying, "I will try to change," and the group is saying, "We want you to change and we want to help you to be successful in changing." This encouragement can be a powerful asset to the member and promotes a more supportive environment that is conducive to change. Because the contract creates a formal approach to the specified behavior it encourages all involved to examine the situation objectively and deal with it more constructively. In future, when the member arrives on time, not only will the successful behavior be lauded by the group but the successful adherence to the contract will also be recognized. Because the group now has a vested interest, when the member is once again late, the group's response is more apt to be exploratory ("What happened?" "How can we help?") than hostile, as in the angry looks and comments ("You're late again") before. In essence, with a contract you have two parties working toward change instead of just one.

Cognitive Restructuring   Simply put *cognitive restructuring,* which is emphasized in Albert Ellis's rationale–emotive therapy means changing one's thoughts and convictions (Clark, 1992). Ellis (1989) refers to this technique as "disputing irrational beliefs" (p. 199). It is rooted in the assumption that one's feelings and behaviors are directed by one's thinking and that distortions in the thinking process can cause negative emotions (depression) and maladaptive behaviors. Therapists of all disciplines are aware of how the "I-can't-do-anything" self-concept can affect a person's self-esteem, resulting in that person feeling "I am no good." Poor self-concept and low self-esteem are probably two of the most frequently used descriptors of persons suffering from emotional illness.

All therapists have had clients who have automatic thoughts of "I'm stupid," or "This is stupid," which hamper their total approach to life. Changing these thinking patterns is a difficult first step in building confidence and capability. Haaga and Davison (1986) describe the need to go beyond modifying these automatic thoughts to determining the themes of the underlying dysfunctional assumptions and then modifying them. For example, the theme of the underlying dysfunctional assumption for the automatic thoughts focused on stupidity may be one of competence. So, by ensuring successful task experiences, the therapist can present a case for competent behaviors. Through discussion of the client's abilities the leader can help him become aware of how the "shoulds" ("I *should* be able to do it"), the "musts"

("I *must* do it perfectly"), and the "have-tos", ("I *have to* do it right") dominate thinking and give rise to a distorted assumption of personal stupidity.

Using the same approach in a group, the leader would select a task or activity that the group can successfully accomplish in order to promote thoughts of competence. While the members are involved in the activity the leader has the opportunity to point out negative thinking by the members and encourage them to watch for negative self-statements in one another. By helping members to become aware of distortions in their thinking patterns and the resultant faulty inferences they make, the leader can, along with the other members, assist a client in restructuring thinking, practice new cognitions, and thus change the way he views himself. This process is depicted in Figure 9–1 and is further discussed in the rational-emotive therapy section in this chapter.

Modeling   Small groups particularly lend themselves to the method of behavior therapy known as modeling. Corey (1990) points out that leaders serve as models whether they choose to or not and so should take advantage of opportunities to model desired group behaviors. Bandura (1971, p. 656) describes three major effects of modeling influences. The first, the "observational learning effect," occurs when the observer reproduces a behavior that is exhibited by someone else (known as the model) but that was previously unknown and therefore new to the observer. This effect could be exemplified by a group member learning to express feelings effectively when before he was unable to do so.

A second effect of modeling is the decrease or increase of inhibitions of responses that already are part of the observer's behavioral repertoire. Such changes in inhibition are known as "inhibitory effects" and "disinhibitory effects" and are the result of observing positive or negative responses to the identified behavior in others. For example, if group member Bill (observer) notices that whenever John swears he is cut off or completely ignored by the other members, then Bill is likely to curb or inhibit his own swearing.

A third effect of modeling is known as "response facilitation effects" and this is the encouragement felt by the observer to repeat behaviors that are already familiar and present because they appear to be socially acceptable. A situation might be one where a member, John, who is tentative about expressing his feelings, sees that another member receives support and encouragement for saying how he feels. Observing this accepting and positive reaction by the members encourages John to express his own feelings more often.

With several individuals constituting a group, each member can observe a variety of behaviors as they are displayed by fellow members. This gives the members examples of alternative ways of behaving (Rose, 1986). Positive

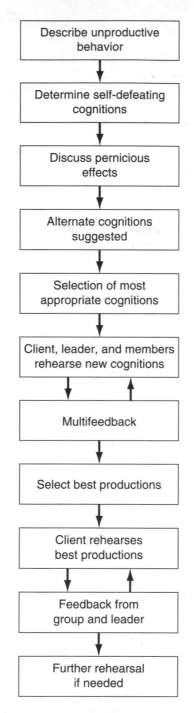

Figure 9–1. Process of cognitive restructuring.

Source: Modified from S. D. Rose, Group methods. In F. H. Kanfer and A. P. Goldstein (Eds.), *Helping people change: A textbook of methods* (pp. 437–469). Elmsford, NY: Pergamon, 1986.

behaviors can be pointed out by the leader. For example, "Ann, I liked the way you accepted Mary's feedback" is an indicator that Ann's behavior was appropriate. Since all members are able to observe Ann's behavior it is possible for them to model that behavior in future similar situations. Because of the significance of the leadership role a leader can have a strong influence on the behavior of group members through modeling desired behavior. The strength of this influence should always be kept in mind, as members are as apt to model "poor" behaviors as they are to model "good" behaviors. For instance, if the leader consistently arrives late to group she is likely to find that very soon the members will do likewise.

A leader employing a behavioral approach in a group may use several of the methods ascribed to classical behavior therapy. Used, even briefly, to deal with specific behavior problems, these procedures can be effective (Smith, Wood, & Smale, 1980).

PSYCHOANALYTIC THERAPY

Psychoanalytic group therapy is carried out by psychoanalysts who bring to the group the classical methods used in individual psychoanalysis. Some of the functions of leaders of psychoanalytic groups as described by Corey (1990, p. 173) are:

- Creating a climate that encourages members to express themselves freely
- Setting limits to in-group and out-of-group behavior
- Giving support when support is therapeutic and the group is not providing it
- Helping members face and deal with resistances within themselves and in the group as a whole
- Fostering members' independence by gradually relinquishing some leadership functions and by encouraging interaction
- Attracting members' attention to the subtle aspects of behavior and, through questions, helping them explore themselves in greater depth

Although many of the methods of probing the unconscious that are central to psychoanalytic therapy are not appropriate for use by the majority of group leaders, some of the techniques and concepts can be valuable.

Leader Functions/Techniques

Free Association   This is a central technique in the psychoanalytic approach and can be a useful technique to apply in a group setting. In one-to-one therapy *free association* occurs when the client says whatever comes into his or her thoughts. These associations are believed to lead to the unconscious wishes, fantasies, conflicts, and motivations of the analysand. When transferred to a group setting, free association can be translated into "speak what's on your minds at any time" (Shapiro, 1978, p. 45). Giving a group this message, with its inherent freedom, can be very useful. It is a means of taking the pulse of the group, of finding out what members are thinking and feeling, what the issues are, and if they are shared. Instead of members feeling confined or inhibited in what they contribute, they feel more inclined to react or respond spontaneously, and in this way the free association is for the whole group. From this input the leader is able to get a sense of each individual, of the group as a whole, and of how they, the members, interrelate.

Interpretation

This basic technique of psychoanalytic therapy occurs when a therapist explains a person's behavior in terms of the underlying meaning. This technique can be useful in a group, although the kind of interpretation that is appropriate in a group setting differs from that employed in classical analysis. It is important, when interpreting the behavior of either the group as a whole or an individual member, to check for accuracy. Laying an interpretation on a group in a "this-is-what-is-going-on" manner without checking the validity of the interpretation or soliciting feedback can do more harm than good. It is best, if you are going to interpret, to do so in a speculative way ("You are all so quiet today, I'm wondering if you are a little angry that I was away last week?"), or to offer an individual interpretation ("Kathy, you seem to avoid talking with Jim. Do you think that could be related to the fact that he is about the same age as your father?"). Interpretations can be effective catalysts to discussion and may prompt members to examine and think about their feelings and behaviors.

To expand on the cautionary note mentioned earlier, if used inappropriately, interpretations can be offputting to some members. Interpreting behaviors or what individuals say can bring about defensiveness and cause some members to "clam up." They may feel threatened and angry at the leader for "reading things" into what they say and for trying to "psych them out." Once an interpretation has been rejected by a member it is best to let it go and try to make your point later or in some other way. Another hazard that can be encountered when making interpretations is the risk of encouraging an extended therapeutic interaction between the leader and one member (Yalom, 1985).

Ego-Defense Mechanisms   A knowledge and understanding of ego-defense mechanisms can help a leader recognize and analyze behaviors and dynamics that are present in the group as they occur. Only the ego-defense mechanisms that are commonly observed in the interactive process of a group are mentioned here. Members may use *denial* to try to fool others as well as themselves as to their state of mind and feelings. In an effort to deal with unpleasant or painful feelings and to deflect the group's focus they will present an "I'm OK" facade to the group. Sometimes a kindly "You don't seem OK to me" will help the member recognize the coverup and assist in bringing issues and feelings out into the open.

Due to the number of persons, another mechanism, *projection* can often be seen in a group. Members project unacceptable thoughts and feelings onto the leader or other members to avoid owning up to these thoughts and feelings in themselves. Giving advice can be a form of projection (Corey, 1990). When confronted, many people use *rationalization* to explain actions or behaviors brought into question. For some it is an automatic reaction, a way of making themselves look better in the eyes of others. By pointing to others ("All my family is like that"), minimizing feelings ("I really don't have time for him anyway"), or blaming others ("If my husband only loved me"), members can disclaim any responsibility for their behaviors and problems.

Sometimes *resistance* is used to describe the employment of defense mechanisms as in, "His constant denial creates an ongoing resistance to the helpfulness of the group." At other times it can be seen *as* a defense mechanism as when members refuse to participate, stay away from group, intellectualize, act out, or talk only about others. Having an understanding of other analytic constructs—repression, regression, projection, displacement, and reaction formation—can also be facilitative in learning about and understanding group process.

RATIONAL–EMOTIVE THERAPY

Rational–emotive therapy (RET) is a personality theory, developed by Albert Ellis, and is an action-oriented method of psychotherapy particularly applicable to group therapy and group counseling. It is believed to encompass a mix of modalities from the two approaches just presented: behavioral and psychoanalytic (Shaffer & Galinsky, 1989). From behavioral it borrows the concepts of behavior change and behavior rehearsal, and from psychodynamic, the importance of bringing internal ideas and dialogues into conscious awareness. Its primary goal is to "induce people to examine and change some of their most basic values—particularly those values that keep them disturbance prone" (Ellis, 1989, p. 198).

A cognitive approach, it is based on the assumption that each person has the potential for both rational and irrational thinking. When irrational thoughts and beliefs predominate and overtake one's sense of self, this results in feelings of worthlessness that outwardly present as immaturity, anxiety, guilt, or more seriously as symptoms of emotional disturbance. This occurs when people worry about what others think and when they believe that they can only accept themselves if others think well of them. Although Ellis agrees with Rogers that humans have self-actualizing capacities, he also believes that they have self-sabotaging ways and that "by rigidly holding their musts they will probably defeat themselves" (Ellis, 1993, p. 532). He believes however, that people can change their ways and can personally alter the way that they think, feel, and behave. Therefore the thrust of RET is to dispute irrational and self-defeating thoughts and replace them with more rational and positive thoughts.

As advocated by RET, this process is a very active one requiring individuals to confront and dispute their negative, irrational beliefs and repeatedly replace them with rational thoughts. A question such as "Are any of these beliefs interfering with your efforts to lead a productive life?" can prompt a member to consider the possibilities of change (Emerson, West, & Gintner, 1991). Irrational thoughts are frequently based on "musts," "shoulds," and "needs," as in "I *must* do very well," "People *should* treat me better," and "I *need* to be loved." RET would attempt to change these thoughts to: "I'd prefer to do well but I don't have to," "People may not treat me as I would like but that does not mean that I am a bad person," and "There is no evidence that I have to be loved, though it would be nice."

A-B-C Concept

One central tenet of RET is the A-B-C concept of behavior and subsequent emotional reaction. Within this concept, *A* stands for *activating* event, *B* for *belief* system, and *C* for *consequence* (usually of an emotional nature). Put into practice this theory holds that it is not the activating event itself (A) that actually causes the emotional consequence (C), but it is B—the belief or the way the person perceives A—that causes C. For example, say a man asks a woman for a date but she is busy on that particular evening and so declines the invitation (A). Being turned down he then feels hurt and humiliated (C), but in actual fact it is his thoughts and beliefs (B) about why she said no (I am no good, I am inadequate, nobody likes me) that cause his hurt and humiliation, not the fact that she was busy and was unable to go.

Ellis contends that people can learn to become skilled in the A-B-C method of understanding emotional problems very quickly and easily (see Appendix A, Session #3 for exercises). He believes that by using this method they can train themselves to stop the irrational beliefs (occurring at B) and can then work to change their cognitions, behaviors, and emotions so that they can cope more effectively with the realities and the unfortunate events of life (Ellis, 1985b). Having learned ways of eliminating inappropriate thoughts, the consequent destructive emotions, such as anxiety or depression, will be replaced with more functional feelings and rationales.

Leader Functions/Techniques

The rational–emotive approach is an active rather than a passive one. It is often educational and didactic. Leaders may teach, ask questions, answer questions, challenge, suggest, confront, explain, persuade, and interpret, and all the while have tolerance for all individuals. Although RET therapists do not believe that a warm relationship is requisite to effective outcomes they do believe in fully accepting clients as *fallible* but worthwhile human beings. In RET group leaders use various methods to encourage rational thinking among the members. Some of these, as presented by Gladding (1991, p. 73), are:

- Teaching group members about the origins of emotions
- Being active in the group process by challenging and probing
- Encouraging group members to help each other think more rationally
- Utilizing activity-oriented experiences in the group and homework assignments outside the group
- Allowing the expression of hidden feelings which are then dealt with in a practical, rational manner

Group leaders, using RET, teach members to use the principles and to apply them to one another. The group serves as a laboratory where members can be involved in role-playing, assertiveness training, behavior rehearsal, modeling, taking verbal and nonverbal risks, and having their behavior directly observed by the leader and the other members (Ellis, 1989). Members are frequently given homework to do, some of which may actually be completed during the group session. In this milieu members have opportunities to practice new ways of thinking and behaving in a fairly safe environment and can receive constructive feedback on their efforts. As in all small groups, one of the most potent encounters is the experience of receiving feedback. To have several people react in the same way and make similar comments about something the person has said or done is an experience that cannot be easily ignored or disregarded (Ellis & Dryden, 1987). It is this ongoing feedback process that enables members to identify their underlying faulty and dysfunctional beliefs. Having identified the destructive thoughts and beliefs, members then have opportunities within the group setting to practice and learn new and more positive ways of thinking, believing, and behaving. This process, known as cognitive restructuring, is shown in Figure 9–1 and is also discussed in the section on behavior therapy.

SUMMARY

The four theoretical approaches presented here are by no means the only ones that a leader should draw from. They have been selected because they each view human behavior from a somewhat different perspective and each encompasses corresponding methods and techniques for altering behavior. As a leader, you may find it most comfortable and productive to function within one framework only in your leadership role. However, it is more likely that on becoming familiar with several theoretical conceptualizations you will find an eclectic approach to be most facilitative. In this way you have more alternatives, techniques, and methods with which to respond to group dynamics as they unfold. There are some settings where the theoretical approach of all professionals is dictated by the director or team. In such cases it is imperative that you feel comfortable in embracing the required approach. If not, you will find yourself constantly in conflict and at odds with the goals and premises of your coworkers. Of course, if you are feeling particularly dedicated, strong, and courageous, there is always the possibility of changing the beliefs and designated approach of your colleagues, but such endeavors are not for the faint-hearted.

To summarize the approaches presented here, the beliefs from which a client-centered therapist works are genuineness, acceptance, and empathy. Through careful attending and listening the therapist is able to convey caring and understanding and to establish a warm therapeutic relationship with the client. The basic constructs of behavior therapy—reinforcement and extinction—underlie the useful therapeutic methods of contracting, cognitive restructuring, and modeling, which can be very productive techniques in group work.

While the main thrust of psychoanalytic therapy, probing the unconscious, may not be appropriate in the classical sense for task groups, the attendant techniques of free association, interpretation, and an understanding of ego-defense mechanisms can be very useful. The principles of rational–emotive therapy—changing irrational thoughts, beliefs, and values through cognitive methods such as the one known as A-B-C—help clients move toward more rational, positive, constructive ways of thinking. The reader will want to further explore those theoretical approaches of particular interest and investigate other theoretical approaches to develop a personal, comfortable, and effective style of leadership.

Chapter 10

Co-leadership

> *It takes two to speak the truth—one to speak and another to hear.*
> — HENRY DAVID THOREAU

Leaders may work alone with a group or they may work in a dual leadership situation with a co-leader. It is generally believed that this latter format has value in promoting certain therapeutic outcomes (Alderfer, 1990). Possibly the most familiar and obvious use of co-therapy or co-leadership is in marital and family therapy where co-leaders of the opposite sex offer male and female models and simulate the family setting. In short-term treatment of married couples, Markowitz and Kadis (1972) describe how the interactions of the co-therapists serve as "parental prototypes" which help the couple move toward maturity by dispelling their long-held perceptions and distortions of parental roles. Secondly, in co-therapy the adoption of opposing roles, such as provocative–harmonizing (Stempler, 1993) and good–bad (Edelwich & Brodsky, 1992) used either deliberately or unwittingly, can at times be facilitative in meeting the myriad needs presented by group members.

As a teaching method co-leadership provides a training situation where a trainee learning group leadership skills and techniques is paired with a supervisor as co-leader of the group. This situation requires sensitive and delicate handling by the supervising co-leader to create a semblance of egalitarian leadership (Stempler, 1993). Trust, respect, and mutuality, essential in all co-leader pairings, are especially crucial to the success of a supervisor–trainee co-leader relationship. Generally it is advocated that co-therapists respect each other, make joint decisions, share responsibility, have similar levels of experience, and enjoy equal opportunity for participation. Nelson-Jones (1992, p. 58) offer some guidelines for effective co-leadership.

- Work with other leaders who have theoretical positions and values comparable with your own.
- Work with other leaders whose training skills and experience you respect.
- Work with other leaders with whom you can have a collaborative and frank relationship.

143

- Share with each other in all aspects of planning and running the group.
- Commit time and energy to working with each other both before and after group sessions.
- Clearly understand each other's status and role. If you wish to perform different functions in the group, you should agree on this.

ADVANTAGES OF CO-LEADERSHIP

Better Group Coverage

The old adage "Two heads are better than one" has relevance for co-leaders. With two persons in the group listening, there is less chance of important material being missed and it doubles the opportunity for awareness of process. If one leader becomes engrossed in an issue or interchange, the other leader, by observing the rest of the group, can pick up on the reactions of other members and deal with them when appropriate. If a member becomes upset or disturbed, one leader can attend to this person while the co-leader monitors the functioning of the rest of the group (Corey & Corey, 1992). As well as supplying more manpower, two leaders offer the members variety and the benefit of their "combined insight and technical skill" (Mosey, 1986, p. 265).

Compatibility

In any new meeting of two people there is the chance that one will not take to the other. So it is in groups. Sometimes a member will not like the leader, and similarly, there are times when a leader feels antipathy or has a particular aversion for a certain member. These circumstances may evolve through the distortions of transference and countertransference (Corey & Corey, 1992) or because of ordinary incompatibility. In such situations it is possible for an antagonistic relationship to develop. Having a second leader who can interact comfortably with that member frequently diffuses what could become a potentially hostile situation. Partners who work well together will watch for signs of discord and intervene to the benefit of members, leaders, and member–leader interactions.

Sharing Responsibilities

Being a group leader can be a lonely and tiring experience. As a sole leader one must be constantly alert, observing, and attending to what is going on with and among all the group members. Simultaneously with attending to every nuance of speech and behavior, the leader must analyze the constantly changing situation to formulate observations into meaningful constructs.

Kottler (1983, p. 176) gives a hypothetical but realistic description of the complex dynamics in a group and the infinite demands these place on the group leader.

> I've got to press Sandra harder. She's slipping away with her typical game-playing manners. Perhaps I could . . . Ooops. Why is Rob squirming over in the corner? Did I hit one of his nerves? There go those giggling guys again. I better interrupt them before they begin their distracting jokes. Where was I? Oh yeah, I was formulating a plan to motivate Sandra. But she keeps looking to Jody and Melaine for approval. I must break that destructive bond between them. They keep protecting one another from any growth. And there's Cary acting bored again, dying for attention. I've got to ignore him and get back to the problem at hand. But what is the problem at hand?

Amusing though this may be to read, to work alone with such complex dynamics is an exhausting endeavor. Two leaders working cooperatively can minimize omissions and missed signals by sharing the responsibilities of leadership within the group sessions.

Support

Co-therapists serve as allies. They assume supportive roles, sharing the responsibilities and helping each other out of any difficult situations that may arise (Gabriel, 1993). This is not to imply a teaming up against the group but rather that together two leaders can offer more objectivity. If one leader is having difficulty understanding a member's point or getting a point across to a member, the co-leader can often clarify by saying, "I think what Joe means is . . ." or "Is what you are saying . . . ?" Thus a co-leader format minimizes subjective reactions, misconceptions, and missed cues.

Group members can at times be very dependent and demanding. Co-therapists can share in shouldering these needs (Gladding 1991). A co-leader who has been the primary facilitator in a particularly tense or active interval may want to take a brief emotional time-out to recoup her energy while the other monitors the group. Leaders working alone do not have this option and may find the leadership role more taxing.

Every leader is prone to doubts and misgivings—"Should I have said that?" . . . "Was that the right thing to do?" . . . "How could I have handled that differently?". The buildup of these questions and thoughts contributes to most leaders having a need to talk or ventilate when the group is over. Co-therapists meet this need for each other. After a session they usually meet to discuss and analyze what happened, how things went, and how things could have been different. This postgroup interaction is a time for feedback, problem solving, sharing, and support.

Continuity of Care

In the case where one leader must be absent due to illness, vacation, professional demands, or an emergency situation then the co-leader can carry on with the group thus providing continuity. However, as with the absence of any member, the overall dynamics of the group will be affected. The remaining members often spend the first part of the group adjusting to and dealing with the absence, thus stalling the movement of the group. In comparison with the situation of the absence of a single group leader, which could mean pulling into the group a totally new leader, the disruption to the group in the case of an absent co-leader will be far less pronounced.

Group leaders will not always be in peak condition on group days. If one of the co-leaders happens to be feeling especially drained, rundown, or temporarily lethargic, the other is there to carry the load during that particular time or even for the session. In such a case it is best for the co-leader to tell the group that she is having a bad day and because of this may be quieter and less active than usual (Corey & Corey, 1992). This serves as good role-modeling of openness for the members. It also conveys the message that even professionals are human and have down days. This can be comforting to members who feel inadequate in comparison with leaders whom they perceive as "having it all together."

Role-Modeling and Role-Playing

Even a brief discussion of co-leadership would not be complete without mentioning the special advantages of using a co-leader model in couples' groups or family therapy. In these groups the co-leaders are usually of the opposite sex, and therefore may serve as both spousal and parental role-models (Jacobs, Harvill, & Masson, 1988). Having a co-leader of each sex also provides a balance of masculine and feminine support (Edelwich & Brodsky, 1992).

In a group the presence of two leaders, who are usually viewed as the authority figures, tends to simulate a family setting. This affords opportunities for more variety in the role-playing of different family situations. A leader, by assuming the role of a family member, can interact with an individual in the group to role-play and work out a troublesome situation. When one leader is involved in such role-playing with a group member, the other leader is available to observe, comment, and give feedback. Role-playing is an excellent way of involving members more actively in the group, of portraying situations more vividly, and of presenting opportunities for trying out new behaviors.

Often clients' problems stem from unsatisfactory and defective family situations. Their experiences with relationships may be ones of anger, conflict, and abuse. For these clients, observing co-therapists, who are two persons in relatively equal authoritative positions, accepting or working out their differences of opinions, feelings, and responses can be very enlightening. Viewing this process of acceptance and cooperation may also foster and facilitate the expression of differing feelings and opinions by the group members themselves (Stempler, 1993).

Training

Co-leadership is sometimes used as a format for training students or others in group and leadership skills. By experiencing complete immersion in the leadership role as a co-leader, the trainee gains an intimate understanding of group dynamics and the role of the leader. The trained leader serves as a model for the trainee and the latter feels safe in experimenting with interventions and techniques because she knows immediate help and support are available (Jacobs, Harvill, & Masson, 1988). Although Finlay (1993) cautions against a co-therapy arrangement between persons of unequal status, it is believed that the training situation is a viable exception (Stempler, 1993). This situation does, however, require some special attention, especially from the leader–trainer. The acceptance of the trainee as co-leader, in the full sense of that role, will depend on how the student presents herself or is presented to the group by the co-leader. It should be stated, preferably by the student, that she is a student or trainee and will be participating in the group as a co-leader. By announcing the role in this manner she is asking the group to treat her more as a leader than as a student. If her student status is emphasized, there is a chance that group members will focus all their attention on the "real" leader, turning the situation into a one leader rather than a co-leader group.

Supervision, which should occur after the group, is where the trained leader needs additional skill. For the trained leader to gain any feedback and to ensure a two-way dialogue during the postgroup discussion, she must create a sense of sharing and an environment of equality. By creating a cooperative atmosphere it is anticipated that the student will feel encouraged to express feelings about the co-leader relationship along with impressions and thoughts about the group. This mutual sharing allows both participants to learn from the experience.

DISADVANTAGES OF CO-LEADERSHIP

The disadvantages of the co-leader situation have been called "hazards" (Yalom, 1985) and "pitfalls" (Edelwich & Brodsky, 1992) and are based mainly on the nature and quality of the co-leader relationship. Kottler (1983) says, "Unless partners can work as a complementary team, much group time can be wasted in power plays, bickering and mutual sabotage" (p. 178). He describes devastating situations that can occur in groups as a result of competitiveness between co-leaders. Leaders competing with each other invariably involve the group by trying to enlist members' support in their cause or position, resulting in group members taking sides. Splitting of the group can also emerge if one leader is challenged by a group member(s) and the co-leader supports the challenge. A nasty situation can arise if the leader has been harboring negative feelings or reactions and uses this situation of challenge as an opportunity to unload previously unexpressed feelings onto the co-leader. Competition between co-leaders is likened to the conflicts between parents who are competing for their children's affection.

Another circumstance with inherent problems for co-leaders is the situation where one leader has a more dominant personality and a strong need for control. The dominant partner tends to overshadow the weaker co-leader and the advantages of co-leadership are lost. This almost always has a negative effect on the group. Pacing is yet another potential area for problems. Co-leaders need to be able to "lead" at relatively equivalent speeds in order to feel comfortable and to be able to keep the group moving in a consistent manner (Shapiro, 1978). They each need to respect and trust their co-leader's competence to prevent undermining and to ensure that each will place value on the interventions made by each other. If co-leaders respect and trust each other's judgment, then when differences do occur, they can be dealt with in a constructive manner.

Most of the "dangers" of co-therapy can be avoided through the careful selection of a co-leader. However, a leader may not always have the prerogative of selecting her co-leader. In this case it is doubly important for the co-therapists to hold informational discussions before the group to acquaint one another with their individual approaches, methods, preferences, and ways of leading. This can be a time to identify differences that could lead to problems and to work out methods for handling such problems should they crop up in the group session. Time should also be spent in planning the group so the co-leaders know who is going to do what and when (Mosey, 1986).

THE CO-LEADER RELATIONSHIP

Most authors agree that the relationship between the two leaders is the crucial factor in effective co-therapy (Conyne, 1989; Finlay, 1993; Stempler, 1993). What follows here are several issues which require attention and consideration by both partners to ensure an effective co-leader relationship.

Communication

To say that co-leaders need to communicate may seem elementary, but the importance of this point needs to be emphasized. In the busy and pressured work environments of most practitioners it can be difficult to schedule time, both before and after group, for talking together. Yet the need for such discussions is paramount for the co-leader relationship to be sustained. A brief meeting before the group enables the leaders to make contact and check out how each other is feeling, both within themselves and about the impending session. This contact also allows the leaders to refresh their memories about any pertinent events or incidents from the last group and to establish plans and goals for the ensuing one. Communication between the leaders will also occur during the session and can serve two purposes: make the leaders appear more human, and role-model proficient communication methods (Gladding, 1991). The postgroup discussion between the co-leaders is crucial and is presented in the next section.

The fact that co-leaders are usually counselors or therapists does not mean that they will always know the intentions of the other or send clear messages (Figure 10–1). It is essential that any communication between the co-leaders is made clear and understood. If a co-leader does not understand something said or an action taken by a partner, she should immediately try to clarify the meaning, whether the communication occurs pregroup, during group or postgroup. During the session such efforts at clarification serve as good role-models for the group members. It gives them the message, "If you don't understand something, you ask." It can also be true that if the co-leader missed the meaning of what her partner said, it is quite likely that some members missed it as well; by seeking clarification the co-leader helps clarify the issue for everyone.

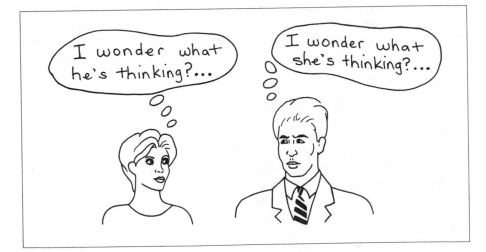

Figure 10–1.   Lack of communication in co-leaders.

Postgroup Analysis

Co-leaders need to meet after each session to share their thoughts and feelings about the group, to discuss and analyze the process, and to note any significant dynamics. A point should be made to examine the participation of each member so that this information can be relayed back to the appropriate team members. As a result of events or incidents in the session, plans may be made as to how to deal with certain members or situations in future groups. During this postgroup analysis, it is also essential for the co-leaders to discuss their interactive relationship, focusing on questions such as:

- Were their interventions compatible?
- In what instances did they agree or disagree, and were these handled to their mutual satisfaction?
- What changes or adaptations need to be made in their ways of relating, either to each other, or to the members?

In short, how well did they work together?

Assets and Limitations

An effective co-leader team is based on the enhancement of each other's assets in concert with downplaying (rather than exploiting) each other's limitations. Giving one another positive feedback on behaviors and interventions is conducive to building self-confidence and a cooperative working relationship. This is not to say that negative aspects should be ignored, but by creating a positive, respectful atmosphere the negatives are more easily given and more readily received. Differences and disagreements should be confronted with a constructive approach—"What should we do about it?"—rather than a finger pointing stance—"What are you going to do about it?"

Competitive Temptations

There is no place for grandstanding or one-upmanship in a co-leader team. The success of co-leadership depends on a "we" approach and, as noted earlier, any competitive behaviors between the leaders are destructive to both the co-leader relationship and the group. Even the simple act of leader A assuming responsibility for introducing both leaders to the group can give the impression of leader A having a senior or more important role in the group than leader B. Remember that the prominence gained by one leader over the other through competitive behavior will cost in terms of the ultimate effectiveness of the co-leader method. The willingness and ability of two leaders to work together as a team is the cornerstone for the success of co-therapy or co-counseling.

Professional Differences

Leaders who endorse widely differing theoretical beliefs, such as behavioral and analytical, are prone to have more difficulty working out a compatible co-leader relationship than professionals coming from the same or similar theoretical positions (Finlay, 1993). This should be kept in mind in the selection or pairing of co-leaders. Co-leaders sharing similar theoretical approaches can more easily and quickly tune-in to the intents of and purposes of the other at any given time. Because of this compatible awareness they are more likely and able to be supportive of and helpful to each other. In the event of a crises they feel more comfortable and confident in predicting dependable ways in which the other will respond.

Now, having made a point of co-leaders sharing similar theoretical backgrounds, it should be clarified that co-therapists practicing different theoretical techniques can certainly work together and indeed frequently complement each other very effectively. As long as they understand and accept the diversities of each other's beliefs and techniques then problems can usually be avoided.

Supervision

Another "pitfall" of co-leadership can be to depend exclusively on feedback from each other rather than to seek external supervision. As with any group, supervision can be set up in several ways (Edelwich & Brodsky, 1992); four methods are described briefly in the following sections.

Blind Supervision   This method, where the leaders describe what happened in the session to their supervisor, is probably the most commonly used form of supervision. It has the inherent problem of subjective reporting as its major drawback.

One-way Mirror   Although likely to be any leader's method of choice for supervision, the luxury of a one-way mirror for observation may not be readily available to the supervisor. This is especially true as more and more practitioners are becoming community-based. When used, it allows for direct viewing of the group by the supervisor so that all verbal and nonverbal messages and interventions can immediately be observed and notes recorded if desired.

Videotape   With the advent of mass ownership of video cameras in the early 1990s, this option is perhaps more readily available and offers an excellent medium for supervision. If time allows, both supervisor and leaders can review the tape together and discuss the group process and role of the co-leaders as they unfold. An added benefit of this method is that the tape can be stopped and rerun at anytime to clarify divergent observations or opinions.

Audiotape   Having an audiotape of a session can be of great value to group leaders for two reasons. First, following the group when the leaders listen to the tape, they can process and critique their performance as well as that of each other. Secondly, the tape produces a verbal record of the session that can be checked in whole or in part by their supervisor. This method also has the added benefit, mentioned before, of being able to stop and rerun the tape as need and interest direct.

The type and degree of supervision required by co-leaders depends on the nature of the co-leader relationship. If it is a training situation and one of the co-leaders is a student, then the senior leader will likely serve as supervisor (Stempler, 1993). If the co-leaders share equal but limited leadership experience, then they might want and need to meet with a senior person as supervisor on a regular basis. For more experienced leaders, occasional meetings with a supervisor to focus on the co-leader relationship can be effective. Certainly if there are problems in the co-leader relationship, outside consultation should be sought as soon as possible.

Resolving Feelings and Conflicts

Although sharing feelings is part of communicating, it is such an important part that it requires a separate heading. It is imperative that co-leaders be open and honest in telling each other how they feel. Holding back feelings of anger, resentment, disappointment, or hurt will definitely affect their in-group communication, cooperation, and ultimately their co-leading effectiveness. Naturally, they should not choose to air their personal "peeves" during the group. However, an occasional disagreement or difference of opinion between the leaders is inevitable and can be healthy both in resolving their differences and in role-modeling problem resolution. It helps members realize that having a disagreement is a normal occurrence in a relationship, that it does not promote a crisis and can be resolved by talking and sharing feelings.

For intense feelings and disagreements the leaders should wait for their postgroup discussion to talk and work things out. If they are unable to resolve an issue through discussion, then this would be an occasion to seek outside help in the form of supervision. Leaders should realize when entering into a co-leader relationship that there are likely to be some areas of conflict or disagreement. If they are prepared for the inevitability of such instances, their reactions will be more restrained and their outlook more positive when the first conflict arises.

SUMMARY

Assuming the role of co-leader can be an exciting and rewarding experience and one that should be approached with openness and cooperation. Whether your co-leader is of the same sex or the same profession as yourself, has equal training and skill, or shares the same theoretical approach, he or she should receive your respect, support, and acceptance. As in any relationship, in a co-leader relationship you need to work together in an atmosphere of compatibility and shared responsibility. Approached in a spirit of exploration and learning, the co-leader experience can be very stimulating. Defining and redefining the relationship can be done through frequent communication and discussion, analysis of interactions, supervision, recognition and resolution of differences, avoidance of competition, and by emphasizing each others' assets.

Having a co-leader takes some of the pressure off you to be all things to all people. It provides for emergencies by offering continuity of care and allows for variety in role-playing. Co-leaders bring different points of view to the group setting and leaders of opposite sex serve as male and female role-models. Taking advantage of the opportunity to act as a co-leader can be a motivating and inspirational experience.

Chapter 11

What to Do If . . .

You cannot create experience, you must undergo it.
— ALBERT CAMUS

Each group session is unique. Even with the same members no two sessions will ever present the same dynamics nor can one predict how the process will evolve. You may speculate on behaviors of certain members, but because the process is constantly changing, individual members frequently react differently given new situations. Therefore, as leader you must always be prepared for the unexpected. Unusual and unique events must be dealt with as they arise. There are, however, some situations and incidents that occur often enough to be considered common occurrences. By thinking and planning ahead you will be better prepared to deal with them when the time comes.

MEMBER-TO-LEADER DIALOGUE

In any situation where a leader is involved, the members of the group tend to look to that leader for guidance. Members will wait for the leader to give direction. In small groups an effective leader tries to relinquish this directive role as often as possible by trying to get members to involve themselves with one another and to assume responsibility for the decision making and overall functioning of the group. In counseling and therapeutic groups members not only look to the leader for direction but also for help with personal issues. This is understandable because the clients perceive the group as a treatment measure and the leader as the person who is the most knowledgeable, most understanding, and most able to respond or help. Other reasons members turn exclusively to the leader are: to impress the staff person with their good behavior or efforts to participate; to try to establish an individual relationship with the leader; or because of their uncertainty about the reactions, responses, and acceptance of the other members. However, for the leader to enter into one-to-one dialogues with different members defeats the whole concept and purpose of the group as an interactive modality.

Members tend to turn to the leader more frequently at the beginning of a session when the group is functioning in the dependency stage. Later on in the session, instances that may precipitate a one-to-one interchange developing are when the leader enters the discussion to clarify, comment, or ask a question. This brings the focus of the group or of a particular member back to the leader, creating potential for a limiting dialogue to develop.

Dialogues such as these are seen as hazardous because they usually exclude the other group members and hence there is a risk of losing them. The other members may lose interest in what is going on, as it does not involve them directly, and they may respond by tuning out. Another possible reaction, especially if your one-to-one interaction is lengthy, is that other members may begin to whisper and interact among themselves. When this occurs, you face the problem of re-engaging the members, yourself, and the individual member you were talking with into a unified whole again. If this happens several times during a session, the group unity or "we-ness" becomes fragmented, resulting in the growth and development of the group as a unit being retarded.

Unfortunately, it is all too easy to fall into a one-to-one interaction as the helper in us wants out and wants to help the client. Feeding into this need as well is the desire of the member to receive what he sees as expert help. As previously mentioned, members usually see the leader as more *knowing* than the other group members and therefore what she has to say is perceived to be more valuable. Now, it could be argued that what the leader has to say might be more valuable and pertinent than what a member might say, but this is not the point.

The point is to involve group members with one another, to trust in the group process for the benefit of all. The members may not be as perceptive, insightful, or articulate as the leader but together they have the potential for dealing with an individual member or a problem quite productively (Shapiro, 1978). Members helping and being helped is a two-way process that brings out individuals' altruistic tendencies. By observing and being involved in problem solving for others, members can gain insight into their own problems and behaviors (Barker, Wahlers, Watson, & Kibler, 1991).

There are several things that can be done to avoid getting caught up in a lengthy one-to-one interaction or to extricate oneself once one has become involved. The best preventive measure is to try always to be aware of the overall group process, including your manner of interacting. The importance of the unwritten rule, "think process," cannot be overemphasized. The following are other measures, both preventive and active, that can be employed.

Breaking Eye Contact

Most people prefer to talk to someone who maintains eye contact with them (Barker, 1981). This fact can have relevance when a leader gets caught up in a one-to-one interaction that does not feel productive for the group as a whole. Try to casually glance away from the member; having lost eye contact with you, he will most likely look around the group in hopes of establishing eye contact with someone else. This glancing away can be achieved without rudeness or conveying rejection and the chances are another member will respond, which sets up a member–member interaction. When this happens, there is an increased possibility of other members joining in. Group members are more likely to enter into an ongoing conversation between two members than they are to enter into an interaction between the leader and a member. In the latter instance members may feel they are interrupting or interfering with therapy if they attempt to get involved.

Redirecting

Sometimes the leader can terminate a one-to-one interaction by redirecting the member to the group. If the member is questioning or seeking advice, then you can say as you gesture around the group, "What do others think?" or "John, how about asking the other members about that?" or "I'm sure the other members could help you with that." This same technique can also be successful if the member is telling you about a specific personal issue. Suggest sharing the problem with the group (e.g., "I'm sure someone here has had a similar problem or experience"), and then look to the group for a response. In this way members are encouraged to interact more with one another, and it enhances the value of what they have to say. You can always make your point or give a response later if it is important and has not already been mentioned.

Members frequently talk to the leader *about* other group members ("I think Mary is . . ."). This usually happens because members are afraid what they have to say may upset fellow group members. By channeling their input through the leader they feel somewhat protected. Members are more apt to talk about another member rather than to the other member at the beginning of a group because the ground rules have not yet been established. If such an instance arises, direct the member who is talking to you about Mary to speak directly *to* Mary with, "John, I think it's important for you to tell that *to* Mary." Initially members will feel a bit awkward or embarrassed by the request, but they usually comply and quickly learn this more direct and productive way of interacting.

LAST-MINUTE INPUT

Not infrequently a member will bring up an important issue just before the group is scheduled to end. This may be due to several factors: The member finds it difficult to speak out but on realizing that the session is almost over, finds the courage to blurt out the problem; the member vacillates throughout the group trying to decide whether to mention the problem and then with time running out finally decides to do so; the member takes a long time in formalizing what he wants to say; or the member's issue is not compatible with the day's topic and that is why he has not had an opportunity to bring it up earlier.

Whatever the reason, the leader is left to deal with a member sharing something very important with little, if any, time left. Depending on the issue and the urgency you might: (1) try to respond quickly and as best you can in the time remaining, (2) tell the member the group will discuss the issue at the beginning of the next group, (3) suggest that the member talk to one of the staff about the issue, or (4) ask if there is a member who can talk with the individual after group and have both report this discussion back to the group at the next session. If your schedule permits and you think the problem is urgent, you could discuss it with the member after group. This last solution, however, can engender future problems when members realize the benefits of bringing issues up at the close of a session. The benefit, of course, is the leader's undivided attention in a one-to-one dialogue after group.

MONOPOLISTIC BEHAVIOR

You will probably expend more energy as a leader trying to get members to talk and participate than vice versa, but occasionally you will have an overtalkative member. Such a person can be a problem for two reasons. First, the overtalkative member uses up so much "air time" that other members may give up trying to participate. Second, quiet members may find the over-participator to be a blessing in disguise. His domination lets them off the hook, allowing them to remain quiet and remote. There is also the likelihood that the monopolizing behavior will, over time, produce frustration and irritation within the other group members (Corey & Corey, 1992). To prevent someone from acting on these feelings with a hostile reaction to the monopolizer there are several techniques that may be successful in attempting to equalize "air time" among members.

Recognition and "Gatekeeping"

A leader can recognize a member's contribution by giving positive feedback to the member, as with, "Mary, you have given us some very good ideas. Now let's hear what the others have to say." As you say the latter sentence, physically turn to the other members, inviting them to contribute. Figuratively speaking, this opens the gate to let them in. This technique, known as *gatekeeping*, can be quite effective. While the talkative member takes a minute to bask in praise, hopefully another (or several) member(s) will respond.

Taking Turns

If you are aware of the talkative member from previous groups, you can select an activity for the session that requires going around the circle and having each member give his or her contribution in turn. This way the leader has some control over the time members have to speak by being able to say, "Sorry Mary, but we are going around the group and it's now Jim's turn." Even if you do not have a task that requires taking turns, you can institute such a process in a free discussion by saying, "Let's go around the circle with each of you giving your thoughts and feelings so we'll be sure to hear from everyone."

Nonverbal Contact

Again, if you are aware of the member's monopolizing behavior before group begins, arrange to sit beside him. If there is no vacant seat, it is perfectly all right to suggest a change of seats during group; be sure to explain why you are making the switch. A comment, such as "John, you are pretty active in group so I think it might be helpful if I sit beside you," is all that is required.

The close proximity of sitting beside a group member gives the leader an excellent opportunity to exert unobtrusive monitoring of the monopolist's behavior. It allows you to nonverbally help the member regulate his input. A slight touch on the arm or hand can be sufficient to deter the monopolist from interrupting or speaking at inappropriate times. A finger to your lips as you turn to the member can gently give the message that he should be quiet. Collaborating in this way is more likely to give the member the feeling that you are *with* him rather than *against* him or *getting at* him. It is a means of conveying caring (Sviden & Saljo, 1993), while eliminating the need to speak across the group, which is likely to focus the whole group's attention on the monopolizer. This method of being beside and with a member will be mentioned again in the section dealing with disturbed individuals.

Confrontation

When you have tried the aforementioned techniques without success or if the monopolizing behavior is very disruptive and you feel immediate action is required, you might want to use a more confrontive approach: "John, I'm wondering if you are aware of how much you have been talking in group this morning. We appreciate your ideas but it is important that others also have a chance to speak." If John relapses into monopolizing later in the group, point out again his disruptive behavior and offer to help him in controlling it: "John, you still seem to be having trouble controlling your talking so I'm going to sit beside you to help you remember to let others have their say." Then move to sit beside John and use the nonverbal techniques mentioned previously. With human nature being so varied, some clients will not be as responsive to requests or suggestions as others. For unresponsive members a leader may elect to set more limits and be more confrontive to prevent them from totally disrupting the group. It is best to be direct and firm, but even-toned and sensitive, in your statements.

NONPARTICIPATIVE BEHAVIOR

There are many reasons why a member may be quiet in group but the most common one is that the member is feeling fearful and too intimidated to speak. Other reasons can be: he has nothing to say that is pertinent to the discussion, is upset about a personal matter and does not feel like participating at that particular time, or feels inadequate and therefore feels he has nothing worthwhile to say. Still others refrain from speaking out of fear of exposing themselves, or because they feel they can maintain their distance from the group through silence. Whatever the reason, it is important that the member be invited and encouraged to participate to help him feel more a part of the group.

Enhancing feelings of belonging can frequently alleviate some of the member's fears and help him feel more comfortable. However, in our increasingly multicultural society it is important for both leader and members to be sensitive to ethnic differences. For some people speaking openly of personal issues is not congruent with their cultural beliefs and ingrained appropriate behaviors (Corey, Corey, Callanan, & Russell, 1992). To pressure such individuals to participate can only intensify their discomfort and is likely to increase rather than decrease their withdrawal.

Given time, the other group members will generally bring the silent member into the verbal exchange (Toothman, 1978). If the more verbal members feel they are risking, sharing, and perhaps exposing themselves, they may pressure the silent member into a more active role. They may think the silent member is playing it safe (Brown, 1992) and feel that this is unfair. They are likely to want the silent member to not only share but also to react to what they have shared. Since the member often is silent because he fears judgment from the others, interest and encouragement may be experienced as acceptance. It is important for the leader to try to engage a quiet person in the group using methods that are not a threat to the member or the group. Following are some techniques that can be facilitative and constructive for the leader to employ in attempting to involve the silent member.

Eye Contact

In any situation people are much more likely to talk if another person is looking directly at them when they speak. Finlay (1993) notes that learning to include all group members using eye contact is a skill requiring practice but is "crucial if we want to communicate interest, recognition, and support for all members of the group" (p. 43). So to induce a quiet member to speak, look directly at *him* when speaking to the whole group with the intention of encouraging *him* to respond. When an opportunity presents itself say, "What does everyone think about that?" or "How do people feel about that?"—look at the quiet member as if you are expecting *him* to answer. It is easier for the member to respond in such a situation if you maintain eye contact than if you are glancing all around the group while posing your question. Once the member is speaking it is easier to further facilitate *his* interaction with others.

Agreement with Others

If a member is struggling with one of the inhibiting factors mentioned previously, a first effort to bring him into the group may be to have him agree or disagree with a contribution by another member. To inquire, "Peter, do you agree with what Mary just said?," makes a very minor demand. Peter need only say yes or no. It is true that he is more likely to say yes in order to be left alone, but at least he has broken his barrier of silence by speaking. Breaking this barrier is the first big step toward becoming a participating member. The longer a member remains silent, the more difficult it becomes for him to speak. Requesting Peter's agreement or disagreement also gives Peter the message that his thoughts on the subject are important and this, in turn, is likely to enhance his self-confidence.

Asking for an Opinion

To continue with the example of Peter, once he has broken the barrier of silence by agreeing with another member, follow up by getting a more individual response. You might try, "Peter, how do you feel about . . . ," or, "Peter, what is your opinion on . . ." This may put Peter on the spot, but with a caring and encouraging tone of voice you can give him the message that his feelings or opinions are important and both you and the group want to hear them. This may offer the encouragement or push he needs to feel a little safer and more comfortable in sharing his views. If he feels recognition and acceptance each time he speaks, this will increase the likelihood of him saying more and of eventually being able to participate spontaneously.

Taking Turns

The technique of going around the circle, with members having their say in turn, also works well in facilitating participation by the quiet member. Used at the beginning of a session it facilitates early contributions by quiet members that can enhance their comfort level and increase the likelihood of their further participation (Enns, 1992). This format is not recommended as a continual way for the group to interact though because it prohibits spontaneity and restricts interactions among the members. During the process of going around the circle members may become preoccupied with thoughts of what they are going to say when it is their turn instead of listening to what is being said at the moment. It also takes away the opportunity for members to respond to one another immediately if it is not their turn, and thus important material is sometimes lost because the moment passes. However, it can be a very useful method to employ occasionally as a way of bringing each member into contact with the others or of encouraging participation when the group is very new or has run out of steam.

Direct Questioning

If a member who usually participates appears withdrawn in a particular session, a leader might ask about his silence: "Robert, you usually share with us, but so far today you haven't said anything. Tell us why you are so quiet?" Be careful in phrasing your question in this instance because a closed question, such as "Robert, you are so quiet today. Is anything wrong?" may elicit only a negative response, leaving you and the group none the wiser. You need to ask the question in a format likely to elicit an explanation; his explanation can then be followed up with further questions or comments by yourself or other group members.

GROUP SILENCE

When the whole group is silent, far greater discomfort is experienced by all who are present than when only one member is silent (Toothman, 1978). All groups will experience this type of total silence periodically and for different reasons. Silence can come at the resolution or conclusion of an issue or exchange leaving the group in a state of "Where do we go from here?" Conversely, silence may be the result of an unresolved issue with the members wondering, "What do we do now?" Perhaps some strong opposing views have been presented and the group reaches an impasse. Not knowing how to handle the conflict, members withdraw into silence. In another instance an individual may share a very intimate feeling or experience. Afraid to say the wrong thing or not knowing if they should say anything, the members choose to remain silent.

The leader must assess the reason for the silence, the stage of development the group is in, the membership, and the level of anxiety present to determine what would be the most facilitative intervention. This situation can be one of the most difficult moments for a leader. How to handle the situation often depends solely on a leader's level of comfort or discomfort with the silence. Inexperienced leaders tend to feel anxious during silence and are apt to overestimate its duration as well as feel a pressing need to do something to end it. This combination often leads them to take the initiative in intervening to break the silence.

A rule of thumb is that the most anxious person, whether member or leader, will make the move to end the silence. So if you, as leader, are feeling uncomfortable, you can be quite sure that some group members are feeling uncomfortable as well. The choice then becomes whether to wait for a member to intervene or whether to do so yourself. This decision will be based on your assessment of the immediate situation. By scanning the group you may notice a member who seems on the verge of speaking but appears hesitant. Sometimes a nod of your head or an inviting word is all that's required to facilitate the member's contribution. The idea here is to give the member permission to speak (Jacobs, Harvill, & Masson, 1988).

A different kind of silence can occur following a meaningful and moving interchange among a few or even all of the group members. This type of silence is more comfortable and may be accompanied by some nonverbal exchanges while members relax and assimilate the experience. There is no tension evident and members give no indications of wanting to move on immediately.

TERMINATION

It is deemed healthy to build the idea of termination into the design of a group right from the beginning. To avoid the abruptness or sense of loss inherent in the concept of ending, it is more positive to view termination as a transition—a time to move on (Douglas, 1991). There are three primary types of termination that can occur in the life of a group. They are: (1) a group member stops coming to group; (2) the group, as an entity, concludes because the contracted number of sessions have been completed; and (3) the staff member must terminate her role as leader in the group. There are also times when a group will terminate because of unplanned situational factors. For example, this could occur if there are too few members available to maintain the group, or if the overall treatment program is suddenly changed. Such abrupt terminations do not allow for preplanning and can only be dealt with individually. The three primary types are discussed separately here.

Member Termination

There can be several reasons why a member may stop coming to the group: he may be given an earlier discharge than was planned, he may discharge himself, he may be dissatisfied with the group and so drops out, or he may be terminated because both he and the leader feel his planned goals have been attained. A member who drops out usually does so because he was not adequately prepared for the group, does not feel the norms or goals of the group are conducive to change, or simply does not personally feel comfortable in the group (Hansen, Warner, & Smith, 1980). Whenever a termination occurs, the occurrence needs to be addressed, because the absence will affect the overall dynamics of the group. In effect, if even one member leaves the group, then the remaining members must re-form into what is basically a new group. This is especially true if the member has been an active member and has played a significant role in the group.

In the situation where a member has been discharged, it is likely that the leader has received advance notice in which case she can pass this information on to the group. In doing so you should invite the members to express their feelings about the member's leaving. The reactions of the remaining members are likely to vary, with some thinking they should leave also ("If he's ready to go, then so am I"), while others may fear being discharged before they feel they are ready. It is helpful and important for the members to discuss these points and by doing so move the group into functioning without the discharged member.

When it is known in advance that a member will be terminating, it is a good idea for the leader to inform the group: "Does everyone know that Joe is leaving us on Friday, so this will be his last group?" Making such an announcement allows the members to wish Joe well and for Joe to say anything he has to say to the members. For example, he may want to comment on how the group has helped him and to thank the members for their part in his progress. Another benefit of mentioning Joe's leaving to the group is to reinforce the fact that clients do improve and in an indirect way offer hope and encouragement to the remaining members.

When a member drops out he may not inform anyone. He may just not appear at the session. In this case, and if the member is still in the program, the leader might ask if anyone knows where the member is and if anyone would like to go and invite him to come to the group. This is a good idea because on invitation the member may respond by coming, and then the issue of his dropping out can be discussed with him. Sometimes the interactions with the other members prove useful to his deliberations about leaving and are sufficient to cause him to change his mind and stay in the group. Even if he declines the invitation to the session, showing concern for his whereabouts can be perceived as a positive message by the remaining members ("Hey, they really care about people in this group.") The members should then be given an opportunity to briefly discuss his decision to leave the group even though he is not there. This allows members to voice their feelings about his absence and to explore and perhaps reaffirm their own need for the group.

Group Termination

If the whole group is to be terminated because the contracted number of sessions is completed, the members should be reminded of this before the last session—"Remember that next Friday is our last session so during the week try to think of anything you want to bring up or discuss before the group concludes." This reminder prods the members to think about the overall experience and encourages them to mention any issues or unfinished business that may be troubling them.

The termination of a group can be a traumatic experience for some of its members. Ending a counseling or therapy group elicits feelings similar to those experienced by a person when a task force, committee, or social group they have been a member of breaks up. Frequently a person has feelings of ambivalence—glad the demands of the experience are over but sad to lose the meaning the experience contributed to their lives. The glad part may come from an increase in free time, a more flexible work schedule, and a decline in workload. This meaning can encompass personal achievements, a sense of belonging, friendly relationships, and a known or guiding purpose.

In examining the termination of a small group LaFarge (1990) perceives the ambivalence to be between "relief" and "grief." Relief comes from the anticipated end to stressful experiences, processes, and perhaps difficult relationships in the group. The grief comes from the loss of the group that for members has become a "living, breathing, personality-filled entity" (p. 175) in their lives. Some members actually mourn the loss of the positive aspects of the group while others may mourn for what might have been. All feel the need to talk about their ambivalent feelings concerning the end of the group but often find it difficult to do so. It then falls to the leader to try to facilitate such a discussion.

One useful practice is to begin the last group with a reference to it being the last session and invite the members to share any thoughts or feelings they have about unfinished business or the ending of the group. Try to plan this last session so there is a little time before its conclusion to talk about the overall experience, what members learned from it, and how they will use this new learning in their "outside" lives (Ormont, 1992). It also can be very useful for your own learning to ask for suggestions and comments regarding the past sessions because this information may be of value in planning future groups. Drawing up a short evaluation form to be completed by each member at the close of the session can be useful. By having this prepared beforehand you will not forget any of the questions you want to ask. Any follow-up procedures that are to be implemented should also be described and discussed at this last session.

Leader Termination

Considering that a leader's absence from one session can be experienced as rejection by the members (Pollak, 1975), termination by a leader is a serious event. Many of the issues surrounding termination of a leader can be handled in much the same ways as were discussed for individual clients.

The group should be informed of the termination as far in advance as possible with the reasons for the change being clearly stated. Members sometimes worry or think that the leader's leaving is their fault: They have not been a "good" group or the leader did not like them. Give assurance that the leader's leaving has nothing to do with the members, either individually or collectively.

It is not unusual for members to react negatively to the announced termination. Flapan and Fenchel (1987) note that cohesive groups and groups that have received news of the impending termination well in advance react more positively than do groups where these factors are not present. Members, especially those who have been attending for some time and have come to feel close to the leader, may feel they are being abandoned. Some acting-out behaviors may occur with members not showing up for group or being disruptive and uncooperative when present. It is important for the leader to acknowledge these feelings openly, but generally—"It's hard when people we have come to depend on leave us." . . . "I know it's hard when things change and you have to get used to a new person". Try to give a positive message about the continuance of the group—"You all try so hard; I know Mary is going to enjoy working with you." Generally, making promises to visit the group or holding out hope of future contacts as a means of softening the parting is not recommended.

DISTURBED INDIVIDUALS

Exclusion of disturbed individuals, such as those diagnosed as psychotic, brain damaged, paranoid, or sociopathic, from intensive psychotherapy groups as Yalom (1983) advocated may be in the best interests of all. It is thought that these words of advice hold for counseling groups as well. Levine (1979), however, suggests that persons suffering from chronic schizophrenia can be helped in homogeneous groups if the leader can accept their lower level of functioning. Task groups differ from psychotherapy groups and this writer believes the decision for inclusion or exclusion of a disturbed client should be based on assessment of the individual client. Several factors must be thoughtfully considered before making the decision. First and foremost is the severity of the disturbance.

To assess a person's suitability, Borg and Bruce (1991) suggest that a leader determine a prospective member's ability to be active, organized, and effectively boundaried. Clients who are violent or acutely disturbed need a brief period to settle down before further demands on them are made. Once the violent behavior is under control, inclusion in a task group may be appropriate. Being included can be experienced by the disturbed person as receiving attention, and this alone can have a tempering effect on his symptoms (Shapiro, 1978). Secondly, careful thought should be given to the type of group or the type of activity in question. Different tasks or activities require different levels of functioning and participation. For example, role-playing requires a high level of abstract thought and can be quite stimulating, whereas finger painting or drawing can accommodate psychotic thoughts and is more calming.

Most important, the leader needs to examine her feelings and abilities in coping with a disturbed client in a group. If you feel nervous or unsure about handling the situation, then, for the benefit of everyone, do not attempt to do so. The level of comfort and acceptance displayed by the rest of the group members toward the disturbed member will depend on the behavior of the leader; they will take their cues from you. If the leader is calm, accepting, orienting, and matter-of-fact with the disturbed member, members are likely to behave in the same way. Having a member who is functioning at a lower level can actually be a positive experience for the other members in that it gives them an opportunity to be helpful, perhaps to feel more competent; sometimes it can offer a new perspective on their own problems. Naturally, it is easier to accommodate disturbed members if you have a co-leader. With the presence of two staff, if a member becomes particularly disturbed or decides to leave the group, there is a leader available to attend to the member individually while the other remains with the group.

Sitting beside the member, a technique used with monopolizers (discussed before) also works well with individuals who are struggling with reality or who have poor impulse control. Your proximity allows you to orient the member or help him control his impulses without major disruption to the whole group. It gives you the opportunity to speak quietly to the member— "Wait until Mary has finished speaking." . . . "It's not your turn yet." Even the interjection "Sh," with a finger to your lips, may be sufficient to prevent the member from constantly interrupting. This kind of limit setting assists the disturbed member with reality orientation by helping him become more aware of his own behavior. Soon the member may begin to catch himself by asking, "Am I interrupting?" or "When is it my turn?" By being close, the leader also has the opportunity of using touch as a gentle restrainer. A slight pressure on the arm may be sufficient to remind the individual that the members are expected to stay in their chairs. Also by sitting beside the member, you convey a message of support, of "we-ness," rather than one of confrontation as would be the case if you were sitting across from the group member.

Kaplan (1988) describes a group which she believes promotes movement toward self-direction for severely incapacitated patients. She calls this group the *directive group*. The group meets daily and is specifically for clients experiencing hallucinations, paranoia, catatonia, severe depression, organicity, hyperactivity, concrete thinking, or loose associations. She describes each session as having four distinct parts: (1) orientation and introductions, (2) warm-up activities, (3) selected activities, and (4) wrap-up. Reality-orienting activities are a major focus of the group and include physical movements, relating to objects, and finally, interacting with other members. Because of the level of dysfunction of the members the co-leaders are instrumental in developing individual goals for the members. These include: (a) participation in the activities of each session, (b) verbal interaction with others around the common tasks, (c) punctuality and attendance for the full forty-five minutes, and (d) initiation of relevant ideas for group activities (Kaplan, 1988, p. 478). Although Kaplan's experience with the directive group has been solely in a short-term setting, she believes it could be viable with the chronically ill as well.

APATHY

Apathy can be described as lack of interest or lack of motivation and may be observed in individual members or in the group as a whole. Leaders are usually quick to recognize apathy by noticing some or all of the following attitudes and behaviors:

- Lack of interest in the task
- Low level of participation
- Reluctance to assume responsibility
- Decisions made without thought or discussion
- Failure to follow through on decisions
- Tedious discussion
- Loss of the point of the discussion
- Tardiness or absence of members
- Slouching and restlessness
- Frequent yawns

Apathy is a mood that can be contagious among the members and can present a difficult situation for the leader. In dealing with an apathetic group, determining the precipitating factors or the cause of the apathy is a first step (Douglas, 1991). If the members are apathetic in their approach to a task, there can be several possibilities: perhaps they do not like the task; cannot see the purpose of the task; feel inadequate to complete the task; or because of familiarity, are bored with the task. If one of these is thought to be a causative factor, then sometimes supplying more information, initiating a discussion of the problem, or changing the task can have a motivating effect. Speaking generally, members may appear apathetic because they feel overwhelmed with anxiety or depression, they are bored or physically or mentally exhausted, or their interests at the moment are elsewhere. Sometimes it is just a bad day for the group and a stoical attitude puts the least stress on everyone. At other times you might want to try to energize the group through some physical activity, warm-up exercises, or a fun event like a game.

CONFIDENTIALITY

The limits surrounding confidential material will vary depending on the nature of the group, but they remain a central ethical issue for all groups (Corey, Corey, & Callanan, 1990b). It is the responsibility of the leader to inform all group members of the norms and limits concerning confidentiality in the institution or facility. Information and material arising from inpatient groups is usually passed on to team members or is charted. Group members should be made aware of this routine. Leaders must be careful not to make promises about confidential matters that they are unable to keep. For example, a member saying, "I'll tell you about this if you promise not to tell the doctor," can be an invitation to a "no-win" situation. By being honest and open you will build a trusting relationship with the members and, based on this, they will respect and understand the decisions you must make about material that is revealed in the group. Discussion needs to take place between the members and yourself to decide the confidential status of material shared in the group in regard to persons other than staff who are external to the group. Clients may come to the group from different units, wards, or programs and they are entitled to protection from group information being passed on to nongroup members.

SUMMARY

This chapter attempts to bring to the attention of the new leader certain problem situations that often occur in any group. It is believed that by being forewarned the leader can be somewhat prepared and better able to deal with the problems as they arise. The suggestions here are by no means the only ways of responding to or dealing with the situations described. It is hoped, however, that the ideas will serve to generate other solutions and prompt a problem-solving approach in dealing with what can be experienced as difficult times in any group.

Some of the techniques presented in Chapter 8 are also useful in dealing with problems associated with monopolizing, nonparticipation, group silence, member-to-leader-only dialogues, termination, apathy, and disturbed members. Remember, though, that each time one of these situations arises it will be a unique circumstance and must be responded to individually. There is no set response or intervention that guarantees success in a particular situation, and all outcomes using the suggestions here will be in keeping with the approach and personality of each individual leader.

Chapter 12

Observations and Analysis

*Nothing that man possesses is more
precious than his awareness.*
— ROBERT DEROPP

The words *observation* and *analysis* tend to direct one's attention outward or toward something and for most individuals it is more comfortable to look outward and analyze the group than to look inward and analyze themselves. However, leaders do need to evaluate their own performance as well and, along with the analysis of the group, it is best to do this soon after the close of each session. If your analysis is left until later, then time and intervening events can cause memories to become muddy, impressions to become hazy, and important information to be forgotten. The purpose of self-analysis, generally speaking, is obvious: to evaluate how you performed as leader of the group. Nelson-Jones (1992, p. 300) outlines some specific gains from this process:

- Identify processes and factors contributing to both positive and negative outcomes
- Identify personal skills and weaknesses
- Gain more perspective on group process
- Evaluate the success of the group
- Clarify ideas for leading future groups
- Gain affirmation that efforts have been worthwhile

Any analysis of a group, and of self as leader, should contain observations and information about the two aspects of a group: content and process. Because group members do not initially concern themselves directly with the process, they will focus on content, which would include the task and what is being said. It is the role of the leader to be aware of and monitor both components. You will want to check to see if the content is appropriate to the goals and if the process is moving the group toward achieving these goals. Your observations and sensitivity to the dynamics are crucial to following and understanding the meaning of the process. This will enable the leader to di-agnose issues and problems early and so facilitate dealing with them more effectively. Observation guidelines can be helpful in emphasizing certain fac-tors that need scrutinizing in order to analyze your group. Some of these fac-tors are: the members, verbal and nonverbal participation, influence, at-mosphere, and feelings.

WHAT TO LOOK FOR

Members

Any person who is part of a group, be it a counseling, social, or therapeutic group, wants to feel that she or he belongs and wants to feel accepted and included. It is up to the leader to think about each member in terms of this aspect of the group experience:

- Does each member feel that he or she is a part of the group?
- Bob is pretty quiet; is he feeling left out?
- No one seems to respond to Mary; is she being ignored?
- John just pushed his chair back; is something bothering him?

Observations like these need to be checked out and analyzed in the context of the total process.

In keeping with these observations, be alert to "subgrouping." Some-times two or three members will form a clique and, deliberately or not, be-have in ways that exclude the others. This can foster resentments and may even be the cause of some members not wanting to return to the next group session. A similar, but perhaps more divisive situation is when a couple of subgroups are present who are opposed or in conflict with each other. The subgroups may have formed outside the group during other activities or leisure time, and although they do not pertain to the group per se, the mem-bers have brought their "peeves" along with them. If you sense such oppo-sition or hostility among members, it is crucial to facilitate some discussion around the issue in an effort to resolve or dissipate the antagonism. Other-wise such subgroupings can have a very deleterious effect on the whole group experience. Make an effort to always be aware of which members are "in" the group and which are "out." If you perceive that a member is outside, try to figure out why. It is possible it is by choice, but it may be that certain dynamics occurring in the group, like subgrouping, are a factor in prevent-ing a member's involvement. In the latter case a supportive intervention may be required to involve the member and help him feel more a part of the group.

Heron (1989) emphasizes the importance of analyzing the overall tone of the group. He uses the term *alienation* to refer to groups that operate in only one sphere of existence. For example, he describes a group as being "emotionally dead" and suffering from "alienation of intellect" when the discussion and interaction are primarily cognitive in tone and focused on generalities and life outside the group. Other groups that become immersed in heavy emotional content do not benefit from reflection or thinking and are said to suffer from "alienation of affect." Because norms can become established rather quickly the leader will want to consider the tone of the group in any analysis and plan ways to achieve a more balanced atmosphere.

Observing and actually charting members' contributions in terms of membership roles (see Chapter 5) also can be useful in obtaining an overall view of the group. Another way is to focus on more discreet behaviors (e.g., Who interrupts? Who fidgets? Who is talkative? Who is silent? Who questions? Who answers? Who is open? Who is closed?). Discerning these roles assists in analyzing the process. For example, if members are constantly being interrupted, you might ask yourself (or the group): "Is anybody listening?"

Everyone's behavior changes from time to time. Each session is a new experience for the members just as each day is a new day. Thoughts change, feelings change, the group composition may change, so it is a good idea to focus observations and initial questions on finding out how each person is feeling. An early check like this can often tap into and ward off the possibility of problems arising later in the session. If Tom appears upset or angry, it is better to deal with it at the beginning of the group, rather than risk that his feelings will affect the whole group's experience negatively. Similarly, if an individual seems to be especially euphoric, some recognition and an inquiry into this state is appropriate. Vigilance is required throughout the session in order to be aware of affective changes in any of the members. The main point is to watch for changes in behaviors, especially abrupt changes, and then, through checking directly or making further observations, try to establish causes and meanings.

Verbal and Nonverbal Participation

Observing the verbal participation of the group members is quite straightforward, but picking up on the nonverbal messages requires a sensitive general awareness. It means constantly scanning the group, watching for changing facial expressions and postures, listening for changes in voice tones, and being alert to gestures. All of these will contribute to a general analysis of what is going on in the group. In terms of verbal interactions an internal questioning of what you hear and observe will facilitate your analysis:

- Who talks to whom and how much?
- Is the seating arrangement affecting participation?
- Do the verbal members tend to take over the group?
- Are the quiet members squelched when they try to participate?
- What are the shifts and changes in participation?

- Do the high participators become quiet and the quiet members suddenly become talkative? If so, why?
- Did something specific happen that should be dealt with?
- Who keeps the ball rolling and how does the rest of the group react to this member? Are they relieved, resistive, compliant, annoyed, or interested?

The behaviors of individual members, such as compulsive talking, scapegoating, and attention seeking, can impede the participation of others. Other more positive behaviors, such as encouraging comments, supportive statements, and questions of interest, can enhance the participation of others. The questions and answers that you generate, either within yourself or from the members, will influence your analysis and direct the types of interventions you make.

Content is also a factor in participation. In a task group, members' likes or dislikes of the activity to a great extent will determine the degree of their involvement. Observations will help the leader analyze the task as being appropriate or inappropriate for the group at this time. Is it too easy, too complex, not of interest to these particular members, or just not relevant in the context of the group today? Your analysis of the situation may suggest that a change or adaptation of the task is in order. In a counseling group your observations will help you answer similar questions. What about the discussion? Is it of interest to most members? Is it superficial with the members skirting issues? Or are they honestly grappling with their problems? Sometimes making a contribution to the content by way of sharing a personal experience can affect the affective nature of the discussion. A good idea? Analyze and decide.

Influence

A member may be an active participator but have very little influence in the group. He may have a lot to say, but in spite of this Tim is basically ignored by the other group members. Another member may say very little, but when she does speak, Mae commands the attention of the whole group. This member is said to have influence. Members with influence frequently emerge as leaders. Leaders, of course, have a strong influence on the group and must be careful to always use it wisely. Their status affords them the ultimate power in the group, but exercising this power, except under exceptional circumstances, without consulting with or explaining to the group, can be a destructive maneuver.

The group as a whole usually has more influence than any individual member (Mosey, 1986), but a particularly powerful person is capable of influencing the whole group. This can present problems if the influence is not thought to be productive ("have a bad influence"). A member may be awarded power by his status alone, and because the other members assume a "he-knows-best attitude," they are reluctant to disagree or try to promote their own ideas. This usually calls for a gatekeeping intervention by the leader to facilitate participation by the other members.

In analyzing your group you will want to determine how and why the members or just certain members are being influenced. Mosey (1986) describes three major ways of responding positively to influence. They are presented here as ways the group as a whole might respond but hold true as well for the responses of individual members.

1. The group may respond to influence because they see the possibility of achieving desired outcomes. This is like "jumping on the bandwagon" to reap rewards.
2. The group or some members may want to stay on good terms with the person of influence to ensure that they are in concert with what they perceive is likely to be the winning side.
3. The members may genuinely agree with the ideas and propositions of an individual and so feel inclined and comfortable in responding positively. Influential members can be key figures in your group and need special heed.

In observing how the group or certain members are being influenced, the analysis should focus on the effects of the influence to determine if the results are productive or destructive for the well-being of all the members. Influential members can be key figures in your group.

Climate

Most people have experienced being part of a group where the tension has been "so thick you could cut it with a knife." Tension of this severity usually results from longstanding rifts or recognized differences and is not likely to occur often in counseling or therapeutic groups. What can occur though, if there has been a particularly upsetting incident within the facility, is that the group members may collectively feel nervous and tense. Other possible tension-producing events are new members joining the group, conflicts among or between individuals, and members experiencing severe emotional upsets (Gladding, 1991). It can be beneficial to check with other staff members prior to the session to find out if there have been any recent disturbing incidents.

Conversely, at another time a leader may find that the members of the group are "feeling high." Some may be excited in anticipation of personal events to come, others because they are having a good day, and still others as a symptom of their problems. Whatever the reason, the elevated spirits often are contagious, making it difficult for the members to focus on the task or discussion at hand. Having observed the rising mood you then need to decide, based on your analysis of what is going on, what plan of action to take. For example, you might decide that doing a few exercises may help the members dissipate some of their excess energy and enable them to settle down. Changes in the mood, especially abrupt ones, usually are indicative of something going on among the members. Observe it. Check it. Analyze it.

As mentioned elsewhere, the leader plays a key role in establishing the atmosphere of any group. If you are down and the group seems down, recognizing this similarity is probably the first step in analyzing the dynamics. Something else to be aware of is that all members do not enjoy the same affective atmosphere. Some will prefer a totally congenial atmosphere and will quickly attempt to suppress any conflict or expression of negative feelings. Others seem to thrive on disagreement and may actively provoke or annoy their fellow members to "stir things up a bit." It is the responsibility of the leader to be sensitive to these differences, observe their effects, and, after analyzing the options, take whatever action is felt to be necessary.

Feelings

When we refer to a member of a counseling or therapy group, we often talk about him having "emotional" problems. In many cases the emotional problem stems from the person's controlling his emotions through defense mechanisms such as repression or suppression (Waldinger, 1990). Often the goal in these groups is to purposely precipitate the sharing of emotions by the members as a method of helping them learn how to express their feelings. For some this will be much more difficult than for others. Feelings are also frequently generated by the interactions among members during group sessions. In all instances of members expressing emotions, observations should focus on the quality of the experience for the member—Are the other members supportive? Is caring shown? How intense are the feelings?

An analysis of the situation should tell you when and if you should intervene. Watch for a buildup of emotions in a member. If feelings are expressed at the time of first awareness, they usually can be expressed in a relatively calm way, whereas after buildup there is a risk of a more explosive reaction. You may start to think of yourself as a broken record, always asking questions like, "How do you feel?" or commenting as in "Mary, you seem to be feeling [sad, angry, frustrated]." However, such comments help members to focus on and think about how they really are feeling and their answers help you to check out your observations and speculations. With time, and your role-modeling, hopefully members will begin to check and verify feelings they suspect in one another ("Mary, did what I just say upset you?"). One of the end goals, of course, is for the members to transfer these skills of recognizing, expressing, and checking out feelings to their relationships outside the group setting. In the meantime, it is essential for you to continue to monitor the feeling states of group members and facilitate the expression of feelings as they arise.

Monitoring is done, for the most part, by observing facial expressions, gestures, voice tone, change in posture, and other nonverbal cues. For example, if a participating member suddenly withdraws into silence, a leader will want to find out the reason for this abrupt change in behavior. Did someone say something that angered Jim? Maybe a comment precipitated his recall of an upsetting incident. Is he feeling ignored by the other members? Did he just remember an unpleasant experience and has this squelched his enthusiasm and interest in the group?

If the feelings of this member are not brought out into the open, his withdrawal can have a negative effect on the other members. Another member, Tom, may think he said something "wrong" or upsetting so may also pull back. Other members, uncomfortable with the silence of two members, may decide that the two members withdrew because they did not like what was going on in the group. To remedy this the rest of the group may take off in an entirely new or different direction (Tyson, 1989). By this time the group is floundering—all the members are feeling pretty anxious and little is being accomplished. This emphasizes how watching for and identifying possible pentup feelings serves as both a facilitative and preventive measure.

INTERACTION PROCESS ANALYSIS

A more formal method of observation and analysis has been formulated by Bales (1950, 1970). He presents a detailed, in-depth, but in its entirety, a rather complicated method of analyzing interactions based on task and maintenance issues. He later refers to his method as SYMLOG—A System for the Multiple Level Observation of Groups (Bales, Cohen, & Williamson, 1979). For a comprehensive examination of Bales's method the reader is referred to his books; only an overview of his selected categories is presented here. His interaction process analysis organizes all member contributions and reactions into three basic categories: (1) positive social/emotional area, (2) negative social/emotional area, and (3) neutral task area. Some examples of interactions within these three areas are shown below:

Positive Social/Emotional Area

- Gives help
- Agrees
- Concurs
- Complies
- Shows understanding

Negative Social/Emotional Area

- Withholds help
- Disagrees

- Withdraws
- Rejects
- Deflates others

Neutral Task Area

- Asks for and gives information and opinions
- Clarifies
- Expresses feelings
- Asks for and gives direction

Bales believes that in evaluating the "how" of the communications the observer can obtain important information about the members and what is happening in the group. For example, if you used Bales's categories and found that a member's interactions always fell in the social/emotional negative area, you would want to explore these findings with the member to determine the basis for his consistent "negative reactions." Or if you had noticed some conflicts or uneasiness in the group but had been unable to fix its origin, analyzing the interactions could be helpful. In doing this, should you find a member who always appeared to function in the "disagrees" category, you would be interested in determining if this member's behavior was affecting the group in a negative way. The next step would be to observe the reactions of the other members to this individual and analyze the overall interactive process.

Evaluation Forms

Using an evaluation form is in keeping with a more formal method of group analysis and most useful if you are observing rather than leading the group. Naturally, standardized forms are more appropriate if you are involved in a group research project but it can be beneficial to draw up your own forms for use in this method of observation and analysis. In this way a leader can more accurately reflect the process and purpose of a particular group. In doing this it is important to have a clear understanding of the meaning of the categories that you include. For example, if you are using the member role evaluation form (see Chapter 5, Figure 5–2), you may find that the category "information/opinion giver" does not accurately reflect an individual's sharing of personal feelings within the group.

Because personal sharing is considered to be an important aspect of most groups, you may wish to include a category under "individual roles" to cover such contributions. You would then need to formulate a definition to define the types of contributions or comments that would be evaluated as "personal sharing" or whatever descriptor you select for the category. It is possible that you may want to have separate forms for task groups and discussion groups. Because the member role evaluation form primarily reflects the kinds of interactions that occur in task groups, it may not be as useful when observing discussion groups. Whatever form you use or devise, make sure to have clear descriptors formulated for each of your categories.

Both the informal and the formal methods of observation mentioned so far look primarily at the contributions and interactions of individual members. Although it is possible to examine the completed forms from these observational methods and obtain some measure of a group profile, Dimock (1985a) presents a method of surveying several dimensions of the whole group. By using his survey with the same group over several sessions, one is able to obtain an idea of the group's development over time. Dimock's survey is shown in Table 12–1.

Table 12–1. Summary of Group Development

For each area, place an X in the box that most nearly describes the group.

1. **Unity** (Degree of unity, cohesion, or "we-ness")

   ❏ Group is just a collection of individuals or subgroups; little group feeling.

   ❏ Some group feeling; unity stems more from external factors than from real friendship.

   ❏ Group is very close, and there is little room or need felt for other contacts and experience.

   ❏ Strong common purpose and spirit based on real friendships; group usually sticks together.

2. **Self-direction** (The group's own motive power)

   ❏ Little drive from anywhere, either from members or leader.

   ❏ Group has some self-propulsion but needs considerable push from leader.

   ❏ Domination from a strong single member, a clique, or leader.

   ❏ Initiation, planning, executing, and evaluation comes from total group.

3. **Group Climate** (The extent to which members feel free to be themselves)

   ❏ Climate inhibits good fun, behavior, and expression of desire, fears, and opinions.

   ❏ Members express themselves but without observing interests of total group.

   ❏ Members freely express needs and desires; joke, tease, and argue to detriment of the group.

   ❏ Members feel free to express themselves but limit expression to total group welfare.

4. **Distribution of Leadership** (Extent to which leadership roles are distributed among members)

   ❏ A few members always take leader roles; rest are passive.

   ❏ Some of the members take leader roles but many remain passive followers.

   ❏ Many members take leadership role but one or two are continually followers.

   ❏ Leadership is shared by all members of the group.

Table 12–1.   Summary of Group Development *(Continued)*

5. **Distribution of Responsibility** (Extent to which responsibility is shared among members)

❑ Everyone tries to get out of jobs.

❑ Many members accept responsibilities but do not carry them out.

❑ Responsibility is carried by a few members.

❑ Responsibilities are distributed among and carried out by nearly all members.

6. **Problem Solving** (Group's ability to think straight, make use of everyone's ideas, and decide creatively about its problems)

❑ Not much thinking as a group; decisions made hastily, or group lets member–leader or leader do most of the thinking.

❑ Some thinking as a group but not yet an orderly process.

❑ Some cooperative thinking but group gets tangled up in pet ideas or prejudices of a few; confused movement toward good solutions.

❑ Good pooling of ideas and orderly thought; everyone's ideas are used to reach final plan.

7. **Method of Resolving Disagreements within Group** (How does group work out disagreements?)

❑ Group follows lead of member–leader or waits for leader to resolve disagreements.

❑ Compromises are effected by each subgrouping giving up something.

❑ Strongest subgroup dominates through a vote and majority rule.

❑ Group as a whole arrives at a solution that satisfies all members and is better than any single suggestion.

8. **Meets Basic Needs** (Extent to which group gives a sense of security, achievement, approval, recognition, and belonging)

❑ Group experience adds little to the meeting of most members' needs.

❑ Group experience contributes substantially to basic needs of most members.

❑ Group experience contributes to some degree to basic needs of most members.

❑ Group contributes substantially to basic needs of all members.

9. **Variety of Activities**

❑ Little variety in activities—stick to same things.

❑ Considerable variety in activities —try out new activities.

❑ Some variety in activities.

❑ Great variety in activities; continually trying out new ones.

Table 12–1.   *(Continued)*

10. **Depth of Activities** (Extent to which activities are gone into in such a way that members can use full potentialities—skill, creativity)

❑ Little depth in activities—just scratching the surface.

❑ Considerable depth in activities; members able to utilize some of their ability.

❑ Some depth but members are not increasing their skills.

❑ Great depth in activities; members find each a challenge to develop their abilities.

11. **Leader–Member Rapport** (Relations between the group and leader) Fill in the percentage who are:

❑ Antagonistic or resentful.

❑ Friendly and interested; attentive to leader's suggestions and behavior.

❑ Indifferent toward leader; friendship neither sought nor rejected; noncommunicative.

❑ Intimate; open and sharing, with strong rapport.

12. **Role of the Leader** (Extent to which the group is centered about the leader and his or her needs and interests)

❑ Activities, discussion, and decisions revolve around interests, desires, and needs of the leader.

❑ Leader acts as stimulator; suggests ideas or other ways of doing things; helps group find ways of making decisions and solving problems.

❑ Group looks to leader for suggestions and ideas. Leader decides when member gets in a jam.

❑ Leader stays out of discussion and makes few suggestions of things to do; lets members carry the ball themselves.

13. **Stability**

❑ High absenteeism and turnover influences group a great deal.

❑ Some absenteeism and turnover with minor influence on group.

❑ High absenteeism and turnover influences group growth very little.

❑ Low absenteeism and turnover; group very stable.

Source: Adapted from H. G. Dimock (1985a), *How to observe your group* (2d ed.). Guelph, Ont., Canada: University of Guelph. Used with permission.

Interaction Diagrams

Diagrams such as those shown in Figures 12–1 and 12–2 are frequently used to capture a picture of the interaction process of a group. Based on the sociometric approach such interaction diagrams are similar to sociograms except they do not include the interpersonal sentiment of the interactions

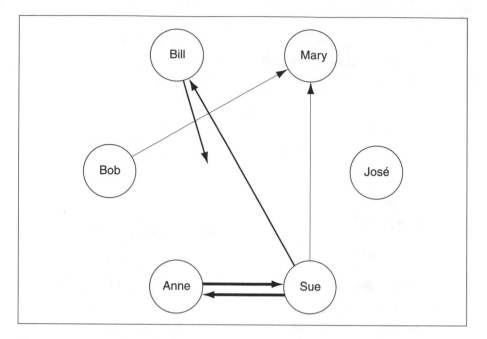

Figure 12–1.   Interaction diagram early in session (see also Figures 12–2 through 12–4).

Circles represent group members. Thin lines depict one communication. Medium lines depict two to three communications. Thick lines depict more than three communications.

(Tyson, 1989). Interaction diagrams are useful in showing the frequency of interactions and who speaks to whom. They show the diversity and direction of participation. Does Sally always talk to John? Does Mary usually speak to the group as a whole and to no one in particular? Do Ann and Don always talk to each other? To be aware of such patterns of relatedness can be informative and helpful in analyzing the process in a group (Dimock, 1985b).

Another way in which interaction diagrams are valuable, as Figures 12–1 and 12–2 demonstrate, is in showing changes in the interaction process of the group. When observations are made at different times in the group, one can observe whether the interactions are the same or different in the two samples. The maximum length of time for noting the interactions in your group should be three to five minutes. Recording over a longer interval does not afford an opportunity for comparison and usually results in such a mass of lines that a clear picture does not emerge.

Interaction diagrams are usually completed by an observer sitting outside the group because it is inhibiting and disruptive to have a person within the group noting each time a member speaks. Each time a person

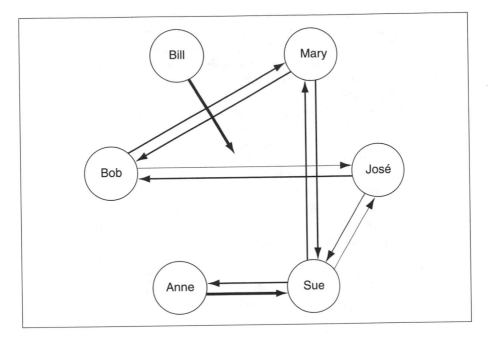

Figure 12–2.   Interaction diagram late in session.

speaks an arrow is drawn from the speaking member to the member to whom the remark was directed. Further remarks are noted by adding slash marks. A member speaking to the whole group is represented by an arrow drawn from the member to the center of the group only. For purposes of clarity, lines of differing thickness have been used here to indicate the number of communications (see symbolic key in Figure 12–1).

On examining the interaction diagram in Figure 12–1, we might think about the following: Anne and Sue talk to each other frequently. Bill mostly speaks to the group as a whole and it appears that only Sue responds to him. Are Sue and Bob making an effort to include Mary in the discussion? If so, she does not respond. And what about José? He is not participating.

Our second view of the group is depicted in Figure 12–2. This diagram represents the interaction over a three-minute period, ten-minutes before the group is scheduled to end. We are able to observe some changes in interactions as well as some that continue as before. Sue has become more involved with the other members although Anne continues to speak only to Sue. Mary and José are now participating. Bill is still speaking to the group as a whole, but why does no one respond to him?

Now, you might ask, "What do I do with these observations?" Well, you can base some of your future interventions on the process observed or you may want to use your observations as feedback to the members. Comments—such as "Bill, I notice that members don't often speak to you and I'm wondering if that might be because generally you look down at the floor when you are speaking?" or "Anne, do you feel uncomfortable with the other members as I notice that you only talk to Sue?"—can elicit important information about the members. Such questions also frequently serve as catalysts to involve the members in discussing the process in the group and the issues raised. By occasionally checking the group process through the use of interaction diagrams, the leader can compare personal perceptions of the interactive process with the pattern that appears on the diagram. For example, say interaction patterns are charted at different times to give two sample segments of a group.

It can be seen from Figure 12–3 that during this period only half the members are involved. In such a case the leader may bring this to the attention of the members and suggest that a couple of the verbal members change seats with the quiet members. When verbal members are closely situated, their eye contact and the interactions are likely to remain confined. If they are seated across from each other, then as they interact they are more likely to make some eye contact with others in the group, which will

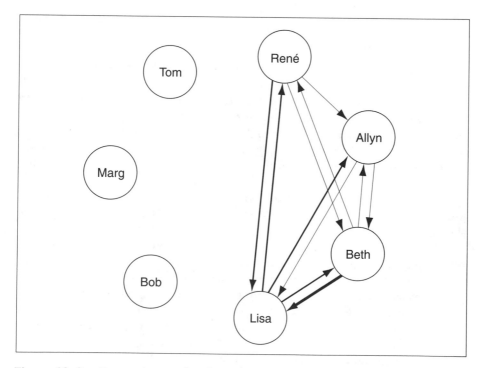

Figure 12–3.   Interaction confined to verbal members.

encourage the quieter members to participate. However, seating verbal members opposite each other also has inherent problems. The two members, interacting only with each other across the group, tend to split the group, making it difficult for the members on either side to interact.

By putting Marg between René and Allyn and moving Beth to Marg's position, you intersperse the quiet members with the verbal members. In Figure 12–4, the expected interactions between the verbal members are shown by solid arrows, and anticipated new directions of interaction are indicated by the broken lines. Because the quiet members are now more in the line of vision of the verbal members, they are more apt to receive eye contact, feel included, and respond. If Lisa speaks to Beth or Jean now as she did before, then Tom, being in between the two, is likely to feel less excluded and is more likely to try and get involved in the discussion as well.

To summarize, it is probable that a leader will employ different methods for observing and analyzing a group in its various phases. There are times when you will wish to focus primarily on the interactions and other times when you will be more interested in the content. These interests will be reflected in the selected method of observation and analysis for any given session.

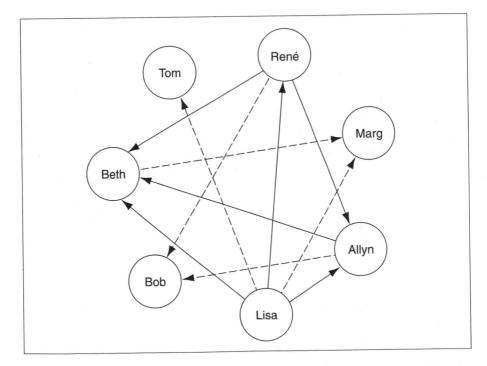

Figure 12–4.   Possible effects of relocating verbal members.

SUMMARY

Finding yourself analyzing your personal social groups can be a hazard of becoming professionally skilled in group analysis! Becoming proficient in this skill, however, is a must for the effective leader. Analysis enables you to understand more clearly the process occurring in a group and forms the basis from which interventions or changes are made. Even when skilled, however, much of what comes out of an analysis will be conjecture and should be checked out over time, and with the members, for accuracy. On the other hand, some observations do glean the quality of information that can lead to accurate interpretation or obvious conclusions.

In analyzing a group there are certain areas that should be focused on and brought into a leader's perpetual awareness. To assist in this process you may want to use a form, checklist, or survey sheet. Such aids serve to remind you to look for and observe the quality and extent of verbal participation, nonverbal cues, member roles, subgroups, influence, and emotional tone. Later a leader may feel that reminders are no longer necessary, but even when she or he reaches the stage of skilled observer it can be useful to occasionally use a tool as a check on the observations.

Chapter 13

Group Activities

He started to sing as he tackled the
thing that couldn't be done,
and he did it.
— EDGAR A. GUEST

As the costs of health care have escalated and the population has increased, the methods of health and human services delivery have of necessity changed. Among these changes are the trends toward increased community services, a demand for a broader variety of groups (Conyne, Harvill, Morganett, Morran, Hulse-Killacky, 1990), a proliferation of self help groups, and a blurring and sharing of professional responsibilities. Whereas task groups have long been the domain of occupational therapists (Steffan & Nelson, 1987), they now are of interest to many other professionals. For example, nurses, social workers, counselors, and psychologists may conduct assertiveness training and teach life skills in group settings. Also, Greeley, Garcia, Kessler, and Gilchrest (1992) note that using tasks in multicultural groups may decrease anxiety levels because the activities add a certain degree of structure to the group experience.

SELECTION OF ACTIVITIES

Activities have been widely used in the treatment of both physical and psychological dysfunction (Bowen, 1994; Levine, 1987) based on the premise that purposeful activity can be a motivating factor to performance (King, 1992; Steinbeck, 1986). The selection of appropriate tasks, exercises, or activities is a key ingredient in motivating clients to perform and then to reap the benefits of their performance (Garvin, 1992; Miller & Nelson, 1987). To be proficient in selecting suitable and satisfying activities for any situation it is useful to first define and then become familiar with the activity. The latter can be accomplished by observing or preferably by engaging in the activity. Part of this process is to acquire a thorough understanding of the innate features of the activity. These include an understanding of the concepts required to do the activity, the number and type of objects requiring manipulation throughout the activity, and the need to or possibility for interaction and sharing among those involved. In each situation the leader needs to think about and determine: (1) what the purpose is in using the exercise, (2) if the purpose is congruent with members' individual goals and the goals of the group, and (3) what outcomes can be expected (Kees & Jacobs, 1990).

Activity groups provide a setting for learning and accomplishing goals that cannot be achieved in individual therapy (Henry, Nelson, & Duncombe, 1984). As in individual therapy, the tasks or activities employed in a group setting must be selected with care and attention. Several writers have emphasized the therapeutic value of clients engaging in activities of their own choice (Howe, 1986; Kremer, Nelson, & Duncombe, 1984); however, the leader still tends to be the prime selector of tasks for activity groups. Before this point is reached other decisions—namely, determining the initial general treatment program, including treatment modalities—must be made in consultation with each client.

Sometimes all treatment decisions, even specific group selections, are made by the team. In other facilities referrals are made with or without specific goals. Still other situations operate with blanket referrals. In this last case the professional will, through formal or informal assessment procedures or both, determine the needs, strengths, and problem areas of the client. Based on these findings the therapist will then formulate an appropriate treatment program which may include assigning the client to various available groups. One of these, for example, might be a cooking group. It is within this milieu (the cooking group) that the leader selects specific activities, although clients can (and this is recommended) be offered choices: snacks versus lunches, lunches versus dinners, items for the menu, types of desserts, and so on.

Before selecting a task, the leader must carry out a comprehensive task analysis to determine if the activity or exercise will be appropriate for the level of functioning of the group members. The type of task and the way it is organized and presented can greatly affect the productivity of a group (Steffan, 1990). It is important for a group session to close with the members feeling they have had a productive and successful experience; they need to leave with a sense of achievement, completion, and competency. Some clients have had limited action-learning, and for them, venturing into any activity or task is risky because they fear the undertaking may ultimately demonstrate their incompetence.

In addition to ensuring success the leader must determine whether the task will enable the group members to meet their individual goals as well as meet the goals of the group. Another factor that is sometimes ignored but should be considered is the interests of the clients (Latham, 1987). The leader should ask and answer the question, "Are the members likely to like the activity?" In conjunction with considering the members' interests, the leader would be wise to also ask, "Does the inherent structure of this activity offer opportunities for members to be creative?" Creativity has been emphasized as an important component in the successful use of activities (Finlay, 1993). The answer to these questions will have some bearing on the decision the leader makes.

The inherent interactive components of a task also are important (Nelson, Peterson, Smith, Boughton, & Whalen, 1988). Some tasks require members to share materials, work in pairs, take turns, work individually, or may even require a single member to be briefly excluded (i.e., closing his eyes or leaving the room). The last, particularly, may be a requisite of certain games but may be counterindicated for some members (i.e., members who are paranoid or who have fragile self-esteem). To summarize, the following six factors should be considered in the selection of a group task, exercise, or activity:

1. Is the task seen to be purposeful?
2. Do the group members have the abilities to complete the task?
3. Will the task be facilitative in moving the members toward their goals?
4. Will the members like the task?
5. Does the task allow for creative efforts?
6. Are the inherent interactive components appropriate for all the members?

An additional factor that should be addressed in this selection process is whether the principal purpose of the activity is that it serve as a catalyst. Some tasks will have inherent properties in keeping with the group's goals. Other tasks may not have goal-specific properties but are selected for the value of the involvement and process required to complete the task. The manner in which the group is conducted will partially depend on which of these two types of tasks has been selected. If the task has relevant content, such as in cooking or assertiveness training, it is more likely that the leader will choose to deal with issues as they arise. In this way members are able to learn and correct skills as they participate. If the task is serving mainly as a catalyst, for example, to precipitate a decision making process, the leader may decide to allow the group to function on its own. While the group is progressing she will observe the process to see how the members approach each other, participate, make decisions, and interact as they complete the task. The process is valuable as it incorporates many functional behaviors that are required in normal day-to-day living. Practicing and learning these behaviors are the primary goals of the experience.

The guided discussion by the leader during the activity or following completion of the activity encourages members to examine these issues and facilitates awareness of individual roles and behaviors. Kees and Jacobs (1990, p. 24) give five goals and suggest questions for postactivity discussion:

- *Processing the activity:* What happened? What did you see?
- *Reactions to the activity:* What was easy? What was difficult?
- *Activity's affect on group process:* What did you learn about others? How did members interact and react?
- *Reflection of feelings, thoughts, or insights:* How did you feel during the activity? What did you learn about yourself?
- *How activity relates to life outside the group:* How can you use what you learned here? What would you like to change?

In the other type of group activity where the activity itself has inherent therapeutic value, such as homemaking or assertiveness training, the members not only practice and hone their interaction and communication skills but they learn the additional specific skills of cooking and assertiveness.

It is usually the case that several group sessions are necessary in order to cover a particular topic thoroughly enough to be of benefit to the members. Certainly more sessions than one are required for clients to achieve meaningful degrees of self-awareness or communication. When using a theme or spreading a topic over several sessions, it is necessary to organize the sessions so that they progress in an orderly fashion. Activities must be graded and selected, in keeping with the group's abilities, similar to the way that activities are graded and selected for individual sessions. Because cooking is an activity familiar to and now engaged in by a large proportion of the general population and also is an activity valued by many clients (Kremer, Nelson, & Duncombe, 1984), it will be used here as an example of organization. The general progression of sessions having an overall theme of cooking and meal preparation could be organized along the following lines:

1. Tasks focusing on nutrition guides, dietary considerations, supplies, recipes, meal planning, and preparations for snacks, light lunches, and full-course meals
2. Formulating shopping lists and outings to various stores to compare prices and purchase supplies
3. Preparation of snacks or light lunches (soups, salads, or sandwiches), eating, and cleaning up
4. Baking and preparation of desserts (cookies, puddings, pies), eating, serving others, and cleaning up
5. Preparation of a one-dish main course (chile, franks and beans, spaghetti, a casserole), setting the table, eating, and cleaning up
6. Preparation of a full-course meal (meat, potatoes, salad, vegetable), setting the table, eating, and cleaning up

It is important to allow time for discussion during or at the close of each session. This enables members to share their feelings and perceptions, give and receive feedback, and generally consolidate their learning from the experience. Sometimes it may be necessary to lengthen the time allotted for a session to accommodate the total activity.

METHODOLOGIC ISSUES

Involvement of the Members

Try to involve the group members right from the beginning of the session. If the leader is active for any extended period of time at the outset of a session, it encourages passivity and dependency in the members. Announcements, if any, should be brief and to the point. Activities should be presented fully but concisely. Complicated and involved instructions should be avoided, if possible, as they tend to confuse and arouse members' anxiety. Even when you want to get some important concepts or points across, first try to get these points from the members. This gives the members a feeling that they know something about the topic or activity and tends to build confidence, which in turn enhances participation. If you want the points written down so members will remember them, or if you plan to refer back to them, have a member write the points down on a flip chart or blackboard. In short, whenever possible, involve a group member!

One technique, referred to in Chapter 1, that is particularly effective in involving members is role-playing. As a learning technique, role-playing evolved from the practice of psychodrama and is now used in a wide variety of fields. Because it is an active technique, as shown in Figure 13–1, it tends to involve members more than passive verbal techniques do. Role-plays can be simple, as in learning the social skills of introduction, or they can be complex, as in role-playing more composite family and personal situations. Other benefits of role-playing in a group setting include: (1) allowing members to practice new behaviors in a safe environment, (2) providing feedback to the players, (3) gaining insight, (4) increasing sensitivity to the feelings of others, and (5) discovering alternatives (Cabral, 1987).

Each role-play generally has four parts: definition of the problem, assuming roles, enactment, and discussion. All four parts are essential for a fertile role-play to be completed. Although role-playing is appropriate in most groups, some discretion is warranted. Role-playing should not be hurried or end without discussion, the latter being where much of the learning takes place. Be sure that sufficient time is available before embarking on a role-playing activity. Members may not feel comfortable with role-playing if there are high-status persons in the group, although this is not usually a problem

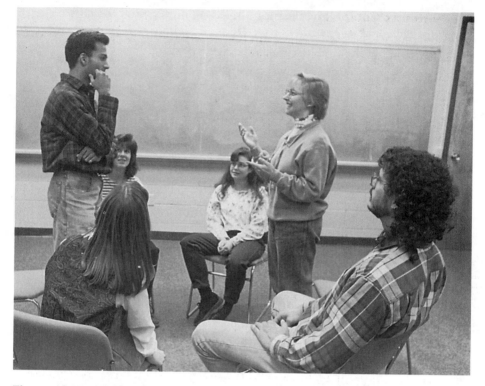

Figure 13–1.   Role-playing as an action technique.

in counseling or therapeutic groups. Finally, if there is only one plausible solution to a problem, then role-playing to generate alternatives would be meaningless (Cabral, 1987). The spontaneous, visual, imaginative, and here-and-now aspects of role-playing all contribute to its dynamic effect.

Use of Visual Aids

The use of flip charts and blackboards has both advantages and disadvantages. They can be very useful for writing down ideas and points offered by group members so that they can be remembered and seen by all. However, they tend to focus members' attention away from one another and in the process tend to set up a teaching format. As this format becomes accepted, members rely more and more on the leader to "tell them" and less and less on one another. Members may also use the visual aid as a means of avoiding involvement by looking at it rather than interacting with their fellow group members. To help the members focus on the group and one another, it is best to cover the visual aid whenever it is not directly being referred to.

Activities as Catalysts

Members tend to interact more and become involved more quickly if they have something concrete and specific to interact around. When using an activity for this purpose, try to have an exercise or activity that is relevant to the day's topic or the issues at hand. This way they have the results or outcome from the exercise to serve as a catalyst for discussion. Various exercises or activities can be used throughout the group as prompts to further discussion or as a means of introducing a new topic. It is especially important to have some sort of task or activity at the beginning of the group that will serve as a warm-up exercise. Members will come to the group from a variety of situations: a protected environment with family, a therapy session with a staff member, being in class, having lunch, watching television, taking medication, being alone at home or in their room, or out on recreation. This means they will be in various frames of mind as they enter the session. Starting out with an activity, even a very short one, is a good way to pull them together and help them to refocus on the group and one another. Attempting to facilitate a discussion without an activity is usually left to the psychotherapists.

Activity groups tend to be focused and topic-oriented. For example, if the chosen topic is how to handle anger, it is better to have the members make a collage, do a drawing, make a list, or choose symbols that represent how they handle anger than to start by saying, "Today we are going to talk about handling anger," and then wait for the group to begin. The concrete production of lists or pictures gives the members something to talk about, and refer to, and will serve as departure points and comparisons for the discussion.

Being Prepared

One can never be sure of the response that an exercise or activity is going to elicit because every group is unique. Even when the exercise has been used before, the same results or response may not be forthcoming in the next group or in a different session with the same group. An exercise that generated an active discussion in one group may promote only minimal reaction in another group. The leader should not only be prepared for different responses, but should be prepared with back-up exercises. It can be boring and nonproductive for all involved to try to carry and stretch for ten or fifteen minutes more a discussion that has been exhausted in order to fill up the remaining group time. At this point a new exercise is needed to re-energize the members. It is important that members leave the group with active thoughts and feelings rather than feeling lethargic and bored. Members are not likely to feel good about or motivated to return to the group if the session ends with negative feelings. Conversely, it can be nonproductive to cut off a lively discussion in order to work in another exercise. The writer has observed therapists initiating an exercise or activity because they had it planned and felt compelled to carry out their plan. Flexibility is the key here. Success lies in not only having back-up exercises but in knowing whether it is the right time to fit them into the group.

Suitable Activities or Tasks

It was mentioned earlier, but is worth repeating here, that the tasks or activities selected for a group must suit the designated topic and the capabilities and interests of the members. An analysis of the activity must be done to determine its suitability to the members in advancing them toward their goals and toward the group's goals.

Literacy is a societal problem that is sometimes overlooked by professionals, but it is an important factor to take into consideration in selecting group tasks or activities. Most paper-and-pencil exercises require reading and writing in order to complete them and so may be beyond the capabilities of some members. This may come as a surprise to new, bright, highly educated therapists and counselors.

Socioeconomic levels must also be considered in the selection of activities. For example, members who come from upper socioeconomic levels are likely to have more money and free time for leisure activities and may see the relevance of leisure or cultural activities more so than members who are out of work or who work long hours for minimal wages. The latter may feel that they have neither the time nor the money to engage in the activity in their "real" life, and therefore are not motivated to participate in what they perceive to be an unrealistic endeavor for them.

The masculine–feminine aspects of an activity have some different connotations now than in the past. For example, where a cooking group was usually only considered of interest or value to women, it is now appropriate for a mixed group or a men's group. Examples of other topics that should not be compartmentalized as male or female are: stress management, time management, assertiveness training, life skills, problem solving, and most leisure and cultural activities.

Leadership Development in Members

Professionals enjoying their leadership roles should keep in mind that group members may also enjoy an opportunity to perform as leaders. Whenever members show some leadership skills and aptitudes, try to reinforce their abilities and encourage their efforts. This means that the leader may relinquish some leadership duties to the members. At times this is difficult for the leader to do because the emergent member–leader may not be as skilled nor as likely to carry out the leadership role in what is thought to be the most effective way. It is important for you to be flexible, tolerant, and accepting in such instances because the rewards and learning for the members can be substantial. This is not to say that the leader abandons the leadership role completely, but rather uses it to facilitate leadership and growth in others. Unless there is an obvious deterrent, it can be encouraging to members if the leader can be open and receptive when members suggest different activities or alternative ways of doing an exercise. Perhaps through problem solving, members' ideas can be adapted to fit the topic and goals of the group.

SUMMARY

Most practitioners are aware of the importance of activity analysis in the realm of one-to-one therapy: Analysis of activities is no less important when using tasks or activities in groups. The same meticulous and thorough process of analyzing and evaluating the activity or task to be used in a group is mandatory. Particular attention should be given to the purpose of the activity: Is it to serve mostly as a catalyst or are there important content components to be learned? The difference between these two purposes have directive ramifications for the leader and the format for the session. If the main goal of the activity is to generate discussion, then you should not have the members spend the whole group involved only in the activity. On the other hand if concrete skills are to be learned, then discussion and feedback are likely to occur as the activity progresses and continues throughout the entire session. In every group, actively involving the members in the process is a top priority and can be facilitated through warm-up exercises, type of task, participation format, sharing responsibilities, and encouraging emerging leadership.

Challenging as it is, the role of leader can be an exciting and satisfying endeavor. If one enters into this role well prepared and with a spirit of enthusiasm, creativity, and diligence, then the outcomes will be rewarding for both you and the members.

Chapter 14

Self-help Groups

*You get help, you give help, and
you help yourself.*
— JEAN-MARIE ROMEDER

A book on small groups cannot be considered complete without addressing the phenomenon of self-help groups—a community resource that has become an important adjunct to health and social services. There are several possible reasons for the steadily increasing growth of self-help groups over the past three decades. The changing health care system with its attendant financial limitations (Green, 1994), where services have become expensive and scarce in many situations, has no doubt been a major contributing factor. With rising stress levels in society (Punwar, 1994) and an inability to find help or support within the system, there is a tendency for some to turn their frustration or anger into a "I'll do it myself" position. As Romeder (1990) succinctly describes the benefits of self-help groups, "You get help, you give help, and you help yourself" (p. xv). The very term *self-help* denotes personal action (Fridinger, Goodwin & Chng, 1992), and in attempts to help themselves individuals have turned to the community to locate others who share similar problems and concerns. These actions are viewed as positive and empowering and overall self-help efforts appear to have successful and effective outcomes.

The term *empowerment*, a catch word of the 1980s, is defined in part by *The New Lexicon Webster's Dictionary* (1987) as meaning "to enable." It is perhaps this process of enabling that has linked the term empowerment to self-help groups and has been part of the initiative that has spawned the proliferation of self-help groups during recent years. Supporting this concept Bennis (1993, p. 84) notes: "In organizations with effective leaders, empowerment is evident in four themes." He describes them as: (1) people feel significant, (2) learning and competence matter, (3) people are part of a community, and (4) work is exciting. All four themes appear to have relevance for self-help groups.

A second possible reason for the growth of self-help groups hypothesized by Llewelyn and Haslett (1986) is the increased sophistication of those seeking help and who, because of this, are more critical of available services. A certain disenchantment, especially with the delivery of medical services, seems to have occurred and the days of "the doctor knows best" and "I'll wait in line" seem to be past. The frame of mind prevalent in society today appears to reflect, in part, an attitude of "I want action and I want it now!" Additionally both the economic climate, which provides fewer services, and the occasional attitudes of professionals toward long-term or lifelong problems, such as abuse or chronic illness, have thrust consumers together to seek out other sources of help.

In addition, our increasingly mobile society has removed people from the circle of family and friends who served as helpers and sources of aid in the past. As Fridinger, Goodwin, and Chng (1992) put it: "Traditional family unit support systems are no longer a viable source of care for a large segment of the population" (p. 20). Isolated, but in need or crisis, people are prompted to seek help from the community and those around them.

Estimates of membership in self-help groups vary widely as do estimates of the number of such groups. Frequently quoted statistics of the mid-1980s indicate that as many as 10 to 15 million adults attended 500,000 groups in the United States. However, Jacobs and Goodman (1989) question these numbers and more cautiously place the figure at 6.25 million or 3.7 percent of individuals over the age of seventeen. They estimate a .1 percent annual growth rate which they believe will raise the number of participants to 10 million or more by 1999. They believe that "self-help groups are well on their way to becoming a major and legitimate format for delivering mental health care" (p. 536). They also note that their estimates may be too cautious if, as others have predicted, self-help groups become the preferred method of community mental health care in the future.

DEFINITION

One of the problems in examining the self-help movement is the confusion of terms used to describe this phenomenon. Various descriptors used in the literature are "self-help groups" (Borkman, 1990), "mutual aid groups" (Gottlieb and Peters, 1991), "mutual aid self-help groups" (Madara, 1986), "mutual help groups" (Roberts, Luke, Rappaport, Seidman, Toro, and Reischl, 1991), and "support groups" (Ramsey, 1992), all of which appear to describe similar if not the same types of groups. For the purposes of this chapter, the term *self-help groups* will be used except for those instances where authors specifically denote other types of groups.

Robert Adams (1990, p. 1) defines *self-help* as "a process, group or organization comprising people coming together or sharing an experience or problem with a view to individual and/or mutual benefit." In a more comprehensive definition Lieberman (1990a, pp. 252–253) says *self-help groups* are:

> Composed of members who share a common condition, situation, heritage, symptom, or experience. They are largely self-governing and self-regulating. They emphasize self-reliance and generally offer a face-to-face or phone-to-phone fellowship network, available without charge. They tend to be self- supporting rather than dependent on external funding.

Katz and Bender (1976) emphasize the importance of personal participation in self-help groups by stating that "face-to-face interaction is a key defining characteristic of self-help groups" (p. 10). Rootes and Aanes (1992, p. 319) add the important point: "membership is anonymous and confidential."

The roots of this self-help movement can be traced to the founding of Alcoholics Anonymous (AA) in the United States in 1935 (Lieberman & Borman, 1979). From a beginning of mutual support between two men who spontaneously reached out to include others, AA has flourished and become the model for the initiation of a multitude of self-help groups. Many of these are universally known such as Narcotics Anonymous, Rational Recovery Inc, Overeaters Anonymous, Parents Anonymous, and Gamblers Anonymous. Presently there are many more foci for self-help groups than can possibly be mentioned here and this very breadth is one of the greatest strengths of the self-help movement (Powell, 1987).

HOW DO THEY WORK?

Romeder (1990) states that self-help groups meet two types of needs. One is the basic need for help when a person is in crisis or has serious difficulties. At such times people need support and need to know that there is someone out there to whom they may turn. They need to know that others have experienced the same difficulties and to learn how others have dealt with or overcome these problems. Rather than feeling an outcast with a "why me?" and a "me only" perspective, a person can gain a sense of belonging from a "we" outlook (Yalom, 1985) which develops from sharing with others in a meaningful way.

Individuals also have a need for independence and autonomy although this need can vary among cultures and educational groups. This need varies too depending on the professional services that are available and how expensive, controlling, impersonal, or rigid they are seen to be.

To clarify the role of self-help groups in the overall scheme of helping processes Powell (1990) describes and differentiates three helping systems:

professional, lay, and experiential. Sometimes revered, sometimes frightening the first of these systems, professional help, has always been recognized as a possible solution to life's problems and crises. When one has a high fever, one goes to the doctor; when one has a toothache, one goes to the dentist and usually these visits have as their goal the hope of getting "fixed," of absolving the problem. But what of the situation when a person experiences one of life's more ambiguous and longer term problems such as a spouse that drinks too much, being divorced, or coping with a chronic illness. The choice, then, is not so definitive and the possibility of a "fix," quick or otherwise, is not at all clear.

What can happen in these less obvious situations is that individuals turn to family, friends, neighbors, or co-workers for help often in the guise of someone to talk to. At this time the person has entered into the lay or "informal" system. This system is particularly suited for persons who initially have difficulty recognizing or admitting they have a problem. Having someone who is interested and who will listen supportively and nonjudgmentally often helps the individual clarify the issues and perhaps realize his or her need for additional help. Some of the more helpful behaviors demonstrated in this informal system are that others "Just listened to me," "Asked me questions," and "Showed me a new way to look at things." It should also be noted that this informal system can be a two-way street—the listener benefits from the interaction or relationship and the helper often may gain satisfaction from feeling useful.

The third, experiential system, which encompasses self-help groups, is based on firsthand experience and offers a process of shared equality. It does not have the "I have the problem and you do not" or the "us" and "them" environment of the other two systems. Self-help groups are voluntary meetings of individuals who experience the same problems or situations and who, through discussing and sharing their experiences, find mutual benefit. Embodying some of the therapeutic factors that occur in therapy groups, as Yalom (1985) describes, self-help groups impart information, install hope, and create a sense of universality. As Clark (1993) puts it: "The peer support group is a very *growing* place to be" (p. 199) (italics added).

For maximum successful outcomes the three systems should be viewed as interactional rather than exclusive. Even if a person finds a self-help group very beneficial, there may be times when the individual needs to consult a professional; for example, in the case of a need for a change in medication or for some specific professional knowledge that is not available among the group members. As self-help groups have become more widespread and have gained recognition and acceptance, more professionals are becoming aware of the variety of groups available and are referring their clients to appropriate groups. In many instances members of the informal system are also becoming aware of the presence of self-help groups and are likely to suggest certain groups such as Al-Anon or Parents Without Partners.

CHARACTERISTICS OF SELF-HELP GROUPS

It is important to realize that the aspects of a self-help group that contribute to its effectiveness as a helping experience can be attributed to the intrinsic processes that occur in all small groups. Much of what is presented elsewhere in this book on small groups in general pertains equally to self-help groups. Lieberman (1990a) stresses that basic elements are present in all groups whether they be psychotherapy, personal growth, or self-help groups. The three elements he mentions are: "the intensity of need expressed by the individuals joining them; the requirements . . . to share something personal; and the real or perceived similarity in their suffering" (p. 259). Specific to self-help groups, Lieberman (1990b) identifies the following four requirements as being necessary for positive outcomes: (1) group cohesiveness; (2) saliency; (3) cognitive restructuring; and (4) diversity of experience. In another attempt to categorize the basis for the effectiveness of self-help groups, Ramsey (1992) notes five specific components as described in the following sections.

Group Identity

This characteristic appears to be similar to Lieberman's (1990a) description of cohesiveness where members feel unconditionally accepted by the others in the group, feelings that give them a profound sense of belonging. Experiencing reciprocal feelings with others creates what Romeder (1990) refers to as "resonance" which in turn promotes identification. The self-help experience offers a place among a group of concerned people, people who can be depended on and who collectively create a sense of identity and community.

Universality

This factor is mentioned frequently in the literature (Lieberman, 1990a; Ramsey, 1992; Rootes & Aanes, 1992) as an important characteristic of self-help groups. As one of Yalom's (1985) therapeautic factors, *universality* is defined briefly by Llewelyn and Haslett (1986): "to see you are not alone in your problems" (p. 257). Initial reactions to crises or problem recognition often include self-absorption and feelings of alienation that may then lead to further recognitions exemplified in the motto quoted in Romeder

(1990): "You alone can do it, but you can't do it alone" (p. 3). Feelings of being stigmatized due to society's attitudes toward certain problem areas are strong motivators to seek out those who share the same feelings and with whom understanding and identity can be comfortably shared.

Mutuality

Self-help groups are founded on a "give-and-take" premise and a process which embodies the sharing of personal information and the expression of emotions. Such types of interpersonal interactions are positive and rewarding but are not likely to occur among strangers. This dual interaction or process of helping ones-*self* while helping others is a powerful experience leading to increased feelings of self-esteem and a more positive self-concept. These in turn can foster interpersonal skills and new relationships (Kurtz & Powell, 1987) giving rise to self-confidence and renewed hope.

Education

This cognitive aspect of self-help groups embodies learning from others, and in any given group, there will be both new and seasoned members from whom information can be drawn. Newer members get practical hints, ideas, new perspectives, gain insight, examine problems, become aware, see how, and get feedback from the other group members (Lieberman, 1979). Members learn how others have handled the same problem and thus acquire problem-solving strategies that are relevant and specific to their personal situation. More seasoned members receive satisfaction from contributing information and also from realizing the gains they have made because they were in states of distress similar to those being experienced by the new members.

Purpose

By name and definition self-help groups are initiated to help people so this can be seen as an underlying common purpose. However, depending on the problem or crisis that has brought the members together, groups may embrace other specific aims. For example, members of AA are in agreement on the need to eliminate the problem behavior of drinking, which is basically the sole purpose of the group, along with helping each other to achieve this goal. Groups that are started because of a desire to deal with a shared predicament, such as a chronic illness, focus on the need to ameliorate or learn to live with a common stress. Still others may have come together not because of a specifically shared problem but through an interest in generally improving their situation and quality of life (Levy, 1979).

Table 14-1. Types of Groups

Subdimensions	Unaffiliated	Federated	Affiliated	Hybrid	Managed
External dependence	Functions independently; is responsible for its own resources, leaders, etc.	Has access to resources provided by higher levels of its own organization but is primarily self-governing	Is subordinate to higher levels of its own organization; dues/fees collected to support higher levels	Is an authorized unit of another sub-organization which holds ultimate authority	Is monitored and/or controlled by professionals
Internal dependence					
Type of knowledge used to assist members	Relies on experiential knowledge, usually shared through interpersonal interactions	Uses experiential knowledge primarily; may supplement personal sharing with information and guidelines gathered and disseminated by higher levels	Uses experiential knowledge, heavily supplemented with information from a variety of sources, including professionals	Uses both professional and experiential knowledge	Uses professional knowledge to set up and operate groups; uses experiential knowledge for group activities such as discussions
Locus of power	Members (or potential members) have power to start or terminate the group, select criteria for membership and/or graduation, set meeting format, etc.	Although guidelines from higher levels are often used, members of the group have the power to make needed decisions	Higher levels set requirements for initiating and continuing a group; they can terminate a group which does not meet standards; members decide whether or not to join or to leave the group	Parents/sponsor group has power over to be in or terminate a group, set membership criteria, influence meeting format, establish governing structure, etc.	Professionals directly or indirectly have power over essential decisions such as criteria for membership; some groups are planned for a specific length of time (e.g., 8 weeks, 12 meetings, cover basic content)

Sources of leadership	Any of the self-helpers can become leaders, often by volunteering	Leaders are self-helpers	Members self-select for leadership, but undergo training for positions	Leadership provided by trained personnel some of whom may be salaried	Professionals decide how leaders will be selected and what their roles will be, etc.
Role of professionals	Professionals have limited, if any, influence on the functioning of the group	Professionals may refer people to the group and/or act as resources, but they do not directly influence its functioning	Professionals may refer to the group, act as a resource, and/or serve in an advisory/consultant capacity; they do not usually participate in group activities or governance	Professionals can function as members/leaders of the group in addition to being resources for the group	Although they may or may not consider themselves actual members, professionals control these groups

Source: From M. A. Schubert and T. J. Borkman (1991). An organizational typology for self-help groups. *American Journal of Community Psychology, 19*(5), 769–787. Reprinted by permission of Plenum Publishing Corporation, New York.

TYPOLOGY

A problem frequently cited in the literature on self-help groups is that of differentiating self-help groups from other types of groups such as support groups, peer counseling groups, psychotherapy groups, and advocacy groups (Ramsey, 1992; Rootes & Aanes, 1992; Schubert & Borkman, 1991). As noted earlier, there are a variety of names used to refer to what are here called self-help groups, and it seems there is also variation in the degree of dependence/independence or autonomy present in these different groups.

Schubert and Borkman (1991) devised a classification that focuses on the structure of the group and not on the topic or problem area of interest/concern to the members. Their typology is shown in Table 14–1 with the processes of the groups being called *subdimensions* and the *types* addressing the absence of or degree of professional involvement in these processes. This classification is very useful in portraying an overall picture of the continuum from truly self-help groups through the grey middle area to classical professional groups. It is helpful to increase the awareness of all human service personnel to the fact that there is a gradation in groups moving across the spectrum from *independence from* to *controlled by* professionals. Whether one type is better than another is not an issue (Trojan, 1989) because, in their uniqueness, all types meet the needs and have something to offer to those who participate in them.

THE SELF-HELP CLEARINGHOUSE CONCEPT

Although self-help groups are now recognized as a viable and positive development in helping people with a myriad of personal and health-related problems, they are frequently invisible to the ordinary citizen because of the very nature of their informal orientation (Madara, 1986). So how do ordinary citizens find out if there is a local or nearby self-help group focusing on the issue of concern to them, and if there is, where and when does it meet, who do they contact, how do they join? This dilemma was recognized, of course, by early members and proponents of self-help groups who wished to reach out to others and make their presence known. Seeing the need to publicize their existence and their resources, they formed what came to be known as clearinghouses.

These early clearinghouses were frequently established by academics and supported by research grants and contracts, in addition, to the work of volunteers and help provided by mental health agencies, hospitals, and universities (Wollert, 1987a). Since then support in varying degrees, depending on the specific locality, has been directed from local and national government bodies to support and maintain a network of clearinghouse activities.

As a result of these developments, clearinghouses have now been established all over North America and even exist in many smaller cities.

Wollert and The Self-Help Research Team (1987b) describe a three-year project to establish and evaluate a clearinghouse as a specialized component of the information and referral agency of the city of Portland, Oregon. According to them, the basic services of a clearinghouse are:

- Compiling directories of self-help groups in the area
- Providing referral information to area residents
- Initiating self-help groups as interest/need(s) are demonstrated
- Consulting with self-help groups
- Sponsoring self-help fairs
- Undertaking community education programs

Most writers on the topic of clearinghouses emphasize the need for increasing awareness of the broad spectrum and the benefits of self-help groups among both the professional and public sectors. In keeping with this directive the following are some of the suggestions offered by Wollert and colleagues (1987b, pp. 505–506) to maintain and improve the services of any clearinghouse:

- Extensive publicity campaigns, including efforts to reach human services professionals
- Callers to the clearinghouse should be informed of its services and limitations
- Calls should be forwarded whenever possible so clearinghouse callers are put in touch with group members
- Clearinghouse staffs should be trained in areas such as interviewing skills, information and referral techniques, self-help consultation, needs assessment, and community education

RELATIONSHIP WITH PROFESSIONALS

Most professionals are thought to have positive attitudes toward self-help groups, although there seems to be a lack of formal training regarding the concepts of self-help in professional curricula (Meissen, Mason, & Gleason, 1991). This acceptance appears to be the case in spite of the fact that part of the initial thrust toward self-help came from the lack of assistance available from professionals and the health and social systems in general. For example, the beginnings of AA, the prototype for self-help, grew out of the inability of the medical profession to deal effectively with alcoholism (Johnson & Phelps, 1991).

Although professionals may be accepting of the idea of self-help when it is presented to them, it appears that their awareness of the breadth of the movement is limited. In reviews of research studying the perceptions and views of both professionals and self-help group members, the main concern overall was the professionals' lack of information on self-help groups (Halperin, 1987; Stewart, 1990). Most are aware of the more well-known groups—Alcohol and Narcotics Anonymous, Weight Watchers, and Parents Without Partners which have national profiles—but appear to be unacquainted with less-publicized groups such as New Beginnings (for people who are separated or divorced) or Seasons (a group for people who have lost a loved one to suicide).

When surveyed, physicians responded that the primary source of their knowledge of self-help groups was from their patients although they also reported that they received little feedback from their patients following referral. Such a lack of communication does not encourage or enhance the development of an interactive process between professionals and group members. For professionals other sources of knowledge about self-help groups were the media and other professionals while most consumers found out about groups from friends (Fridinger, Goodwin, & Chng, 1992).

ROLE OF THE PROFESSIONAL

Because the relationship between professionals and the self-help movement in general appears to be somewhat ambiguous and tenuous, efforts by professionals to approach or contact specific groups must be made with thought, sensitivity, and great care. Probably the most important first step for professionals to take is to thoroughly familiarize themselves with the many aspects of the self-help group movement, including its evolution, the broad spectrum of problem areas addressed, the variety of structural and ideological formats, the different types of activities, and the extent of available groups in the professional's local environment (Emerick, 1990).

Borkman (1990) cautions professionals against attempting to assume leadership roles and emphasizes the need for professionals to respect the group's autonomy and shared equality. He goes on to state that self-help groups "should be taught to professionals as member-owned, self-determining, voluntary associations" (p. 330). It is imperative for professionals to remove themselves from any superior stance, such as that of "expert," and assume a more collegial and interactive role. This is not a comfortable change even for students training in the professions because they have been socialized to think in terms of being or becoming skilled experts. What roles then should they assume in working with self-help groups?

Among suggested roles for professionals when interacting with these groups are those of sponsor, organizer, planner, advisor, facilitator, guest speaker, consultant, and referral source (Meissen, Mason, & Gleason, 1991). A survey of professional perceptions added the roles of initiator, trainer, and linking agent (Stewart, 1990). The professional role most supported and desired by group members was that of consultant. Both Schwartzben (1992) and Krupnick, Rowland, Goldberg, and Daniel (1993) describe support groups where professionals organized the groups initially but then served as resource persons or consultants. In these roles they assisted the members with defining goals, establishing a group structure, obtaining information, and encouraging leadership responsibilities among the members.

LEADERSHIP

The problems in conducting research on self-help groups have been well documented (Chesler, 1991; Goldklang, 1991; Powell & Cameron, 1991; Tebes & Kraemer, 1991). Because of this, information regarding the role and efficacy of leadership in self-help groups is sparse and lacking in documentation. In attempting to find out what mutual-aid groups do and in efforts to focus on assessment and leadership training, Paine, Suarez-Balcazar, Fawcett, and Borck-Jameson (1992) contacted twenty groups and had only two groups agree to participate in their study.

The only criteria for leadership of a self-help group often is personal experience with the problem of concern to the group. Group members appear to feel comfortable with a leader who will self-disclose and who can share firsthand comparable experiences with them. Sometimes leadership is automatically assumed by or conferred on the person who initiates it or is seen as being responsible for the organization of the group (Revenson & Cassel, 1991). In other instances leadership is shared or is passed from one member to another as the group continues and more senior, experienced members are available (Schwartzben, 1992).

As for trained leaders, some feel that the presence of such individuals allows group members to abdicate their responsibility for their own problems and for the success of the group. In addition, professional co-optation is feared; a trained leader may place expectations, principles, or beliefs on the group in an autocratic manner that does not allow the customary, shared, self-help process from occuring (Adams, 1990). Conversely, the lack of a trained leader may result in a negative experience for members because of the formation of cliques, domination by subgroups, and lack of guidance and equal attention to all members' concerns (Block & Llewelyn, 1987). For the most part each self-help group works out its own leadership issues according to the needs and desires of the membership.

SUMMARY

The self-help movement is growing and expanding and now represents many disease categories and most types of chronic illness. Possible reasons for this expansion are: (1) disenchantment with the health and social services available, (2) frustration that services often are not available, (3) increased sophistication and "empowerment" of help seekers, and (4) lack of traditional support systems. Self-help groups are formed by individuals who share a common problem, concern, or situation and believe that in meeting with each other to discuss shared issues they can help themselves and in the process help others.

Groups may differ by name; however, they tend to have similar characteristics such as group identity, universality, mutuality, a common purpose, and an educational component. Variations in degrees of independence present differences in format, structure, leadership, and autonomy in and among groups. Although there is obvious sensitivity about what is perceived as professional interference, it is believed that professionals can have helpful and interactive relationships with self-help groups. Positive roles that professionals can assume vis-à-vis self-help groups are sponsor, organizer, planner, advisor, facilitator, speaker, and referral source, with the most accepted role being that of consultant.

Bibliography

Adams, R. (1990). *Self-help, social work and empowerment*. London: Macmillan

Alcoholics Anonymous World Service (1984). *'Pass it on': The story of Bill Wilson and how the A.A. message reached the world*. New York: Author.

Alderfer, C. P. (1990). Staff authority and leadership in experiential groups. In J. Gillette & M. McCollom (Eds.), *Groups in context* (pp. 252–275). Reading, MA: Addison-Wesley.

Allport, F. H. (1920). The influence of the group upon association and thought. *Journal of Experimental Psychology, 3*, 159–182.

Andrews, P. H. (1992). Sex and gender differences in group communication. *Small Group Research, 23*, 74–94.

Bales, R. F. (1950). *Interaction process analysis: A method for the study of small groups*. Cambridge, MA: Addison-Wesley.

Bales, R. F. (1970). *Personality and interpersonal behaviour*. New York: Holt, Rinehart & Winston.

Bales, R. F., Cohen, S. P., & Williamson, S. A. (1979). *SYMLOG: A system for the multiple level observation of groups*. New York: Free Press.

Bandura, A. (1971). Psychotherapy based upon modeling principles. In A. E. Bergin & S. L. Garfield (Eds.), *Handbook of psychotherapy and behavior change: An empirical analysis* (pp. 653–708). New York: John Wiley and Sons.

Banning, M. R., & Nelson, D. L. (1987). The effects of activity-elicited humor and group structure on group cohesion and affective responses. *American Journal of Occupational Therapy, 41*, 510–514.

Barker, L. L. (1981). *Communication* (2d ed.). Englewood Cliffs, NJ: Prentice-Hall.

Barker, L. L., Wahlers, K. J., Watson, K. W., & Kibler, R. J. (1991). *Groups in process, an introduction to small group communication* (4th ed.). Englewood Cliffs, NJ: Prentice-Hall.

Barrett-Lennard, G. T. (1988). Listening. *Person-Centered Review, 3*, 410–425.

Barris, R. (1982). Environmental interactions: An extension of the model of occupation. *American Journal of Occupational Therapy, 36*, 637–644.

Barris, R., & Kielhofner, G. (1986). Beliefs, perspectives, and activities of psychosocial occupational therapy. *American Journal of Occupational Therapy, 40*, 535–541.

Bass, B. M. (1981). *Stodgill's handbook of leadership*. New York: Macmillan.

Battegay, R. (1986). People in groups: Dynamic and therapeutic aspects. *Group, 10*, 131–148.

Benne, K. D., & Sheats, P. (1948). Functional roles of group members. *Journal of Social Issues, 4*, 41–49.

Bennis, W. (1993). *An invented life: Reflections on leadership and change*. Reading, MA: Addison-Wesley.

Bennis, W. G., & Shepard, H. A. (1978). A theory of group development. In L. P. Bradford (Ed.), *Group development* (2d ed.) (pp. 13–35). San Diego: University Associates.

Berman-Rossi, T. (1992). Empowering groups through understanding stages of group development. *Social Work with Groups, 15*, 239–255.

Berman-Rossi, T. (1993). The tasks and skills of the social worker across stages of group development. *Social Work with Groups, 16*, 69–81.

Bion, W. R. (1961). *Experience in groups*. New York: Basic Books.

Blatner, A. (1989). Psychodrama. In R. J. Corsini & D. Wedding (Eds.), *Current Psychotherapies* (4th ed.) (pp. 561–571). Itasca, IL: F. E. Peacock.

Bloch, S., Browning, S, & McGrath, G. (1983). Humour in group psychotherapy. *British Journal of Medical Psychology, 56*, 89–97.

Block, S., & Crouch, E. (1985). *Therapeutic factors in group psychotherapy*. Oxford, England: Oxford University Press.

Block, S., Crouch, E., & Reibstein, J. (1981). Therapeutic factors in group psychotherapy. *Archives of General Psychiatry, 38*, 519–526.

Block, E., & Llewelyn, S. (1987). Leadership skills and helpful factors in self-help groups. *British Journal of Guidance and Counselling, 15*, 257–270.

Bonner, H. (1959). *Group dynamics: Principles and applications*. New York: Ronald Press.

Bonney, W. C., Randall, D. A., Jr., & Cleveland, J. D. (1986). An analysis of client-perceived curative factors in a therapy group of former incest victims. *Small Group Behavior, 17*, 303–321.

Borg, B., & Bruce, M. A. (1991). *The group system*. Thorofare, NJ: Slack.

Borkman, T. (1990). Self-help groups at the turning point: Emerging egalitarian alliances with the formal health care system? *American Journal of Community Psychology, 18*, 321–332.

Bowen, R. E. (1994). The use of occupational therapists in independent living programs. *American Journal of Occupational Therapy, 48*, 105–112.

Braaten, L. J. (1974/1975). Developmental phases of encounter groups and related intensive groups: A critiacl review of models and a new proposal. *Interpersonal Development, 5*, 112–129.

Braaten, L. J. (1991). Group cohesion: A new multidimensional model. *Group, 15*, 39–53.

Bradlee, L. (1984). The use of groups in short-term psychiatric settings. *Occupational Therapy in Mental Health, 4*, 47–57.

Brandler, S., & Roman, C. P. (1991). *Group work: Skills and strategies for effective interventions*. Binghampton, NY: Haworth Press.

Brilhart, J. K. (1974). *Effective group discussion*. Dubuque, IA: Wm. C. Brown.

Brown, L. N. (1993). Group work and the environment: A systems approach. *Social Work with Groups, 16*, 83–95.

Brown, N. W. (1992). *Teaching group dynamics: Process and practice*. Westport, CT: Praeger.

Buchanan, D. C. (1978). Group therapy for chronic physically ill patients. *Psychosomatics, 19*, 425–431.

Budman, S. H., Soldz, S., Demby, A., Davis, M., & Merry, J. (1993). What is cohesiveness: An empirical examination. *Small Group Research, 24*, 199–215.

Burgoon, M., Heston, J. K., & McCroskey, J. (1974). *Small group communication: A functional approach*. New York: Holt, Rinehart & Winston.

Burnard, P. (1992). *Effective communication skills for health professionals*. London: Chapman & Hall.

Cabral, R. J. (1987). Role playing as a group intervention. *Small Group Behavior, 18*, 470–482.

Campbell, L. F. (1992). An interview with Arthur M. Horne. *Journal for Specialists in Group Work, 17*, 131–143.

Checkland, P. (1981). *Systems thinking, systems practice*. New York: John Wiley & Sons.

Chesler, M. A. (1991). Participatory action research with self-help groups: An alternative paradigm for inquiry and action. *American Journal of Community Psychology, 19*, 757–768.

Clark, A. J. (1989). Questions in group counseling. *Journal for Specialists in Group Work, 14*, 121–124.

Clark, A. J. (1992). Defense mechanisms in group counseling. *Journal for Specialists in Group Work. 17*, 151–160.

Clark, P. (1993). What's a nice editor like you doing in a place like this? *Psychosocial Rehabilitation Journal, 17*, 197–199.

Cohen, S. G. (1990). Hilltop Hospital top management group. In J. R. Hackman (Ed.), *Groups that work (and those that don't)* (pp. 56–77). San Francisco: Jossey-Bass.

Comrey, A. L., & Staats, C. K. (1955). Group performance in a cognitive task. *Journal of Applied Psychology, 39*, 354–356.

Conyne, R. K. (1989). *How personal growth and task groups work*. Newbury Park, CA: Sage.

Conyne, R. K., Harvill, R. L., Morganett, R. S., Morran, D. K., & Hulse-Killacky, D. (1990). Effective group leadership: Continuing the search for greater clarity and understanding. *Journal for Specialists in Group Work, 15*, 30–36.

Cooper, J. B., & McGaugh, J. L. (1969). Leadership. In C. A. Gibb (Ed.), *Leadership*. Harmondsworth, U.K.: Penguin Books.

Corey, G. (1990). *Theory and practice of group counseling* (3d ed.). Pacific Grove, CA: Brooks/Cole.

Corey, G., & Corey, M. S. (1992). *Groups: Process and practice* (4th ed.). Pacific Grove, CA: Brooks/Cole.

Corey, G., Corey, M. S., & Callanan, P. (1990a). Role of group leader's values in group counseling. *Journal for Specialists in Group Work, 15*, 68–74.

Corey, G., Corey, M. S., & Callanan, P. (1990b). *Issues and ethics in the helping professions* (3d ed.). Pacific Grove, CA: Brooks/Cole.

Corey, G., Corey, M., Callanan, P., & Russell, J. M. (1992). *Group techniques* (3d ed.). Pacific Grove, CA: Brooks/Cole

Corsini, R. J., & Wedding, D. (1989). *Current psychotherapies* (4th ed.). Itasca, IL: Peacock.

Cunningham, L. L., & Carol, L. N. (1986). Leaders and leadership: 1985 and beyond. *Proceedings of Symposium, Occupational Therapy Education: Target 2000*. Rockville, MD: American Occupational Therapy Association.

Davies, P. L., & Gavin, W. J. (1994). Comparison of individual and group/consultation treatment methods for preschool children with developmental delays. *American Journal of Occupational Therapy, 48*, 155–161.

De Pree, M. (1987). *Leadership is an art*. East Lansing, MI: Michigan State University Press.

Dimock, H. G. (1985a). *How to observe your group* (2d ed.). Guelph, Ont., Canada: University of Guelph.

Dimock, H. G. (1985b). *How to analyze and evaluate group growth* (2d ed.). Guelph, Ont., Canada: University of Guelph.

Dimock, H. G. (1985c). *Planning group development* (2d ed.). Guelph, Ont., Canada: University of Guelph.

Donohue, M. (1982). Designing activities to develop a women's identification group. *Occupational Therapy in Mental Health, 2*, 1–19.

Douglas, T. (1991). *A handbook of common groupwork problems*. London: Routledge.

Dunn, W., Brown, C., & McGuigan, A. (1994). The ecology of human performance: A framework for considering the effect of context. *American Journal of Occupational Therapy, 48*, 595–607.

Dusay, J. M., & Dusay, K. M. (1989). Transactional analysis. In R. J. Corsini & D. Wedding (Eds.), *Current psychotherapies* (4th ed.) (pp. 405–453). Itasca, IL: F. E. Peacock.

Edelwich, J., & Brodsky, A. (1992). *Group counseling for the resistant client*. New York: Lexington Books.

Egan, G. (1976). *Interpersonal living*. Monterey, CA: Brooks/Cole.

Egan, G. (1983). Some suggested rules for confrontation. In H. H. Blumberg, A. P. Hare, V. Kent, & M. F. Davies (Eds.), *Small groups and social interaction* (pp. 237–238). New York: John Wiley & Sons.

Ehrenberg, D. B. (1991). Playfulness and humor in the psychoanalytic relationship. *Group, 15*, 225–233.

Ellis, A. (1985b). Expanding the ABCs of rational–emotive therapy. In M. Mahoney & A. Freeman (Eds.), *Cognition and psychotherapy* (pp. 313–323). New York: Plenum.

Ellis, A. (1989). Rational-Emotive therapy. In R. J. Corsini & D. Wedding (Eds.), *Current psychotherapies* (4th ed.) (pp. 197–238). Itasca, IL: F. E. Peacock.

Ellis, A. (1993). Constructivism and Rational-Emotive therapy: A critique of Richard Wessler's critique. *Psychotherapy, 30*, 531–532.

Ellis, A., & Dryden, W. (1987). *The practice of rational–emotive therapy*. New York: Springer.

Ellis, R. J., & Cronshaw, S. F. (1992). Self-monitoring and leader emergence: A test of moderator effects. *Small Group Research, 23*, 113–129.

Emerson, P., West, J. D., & Gintner, G. G. (1991). An adlerian perspective on cognitive restructuring and treating depression. *Journal of Cognitive Psychotherapy: An International Quarterly, 5*, 41–52.

Emerick, R. E. (1990). Self-help groups for former patients: Relations with mental health professionals. *Hospital and Community Psychiatry, 41*, 401–407.

Enns, C. Z. (1992). Self-esteem groups: A synthesis of consciousness-raising and assertiveness training. *Journal of Counseling & Development, 71*, 7–13.

Erickson, R. C. (1986). Heterogeneous groups: A legitimate alternative. *Group, 10*, 21–26.

Erikson, E. H. (1963). *Childhood and society* (2d ed.). New York: Norton

Evans, C. R., & Dion, K. L. (1991). Group cohesion and performance: A meta analysis. *Small Group Research, 22*, 175–186.

Falk-Kessler, J., Momich, C., & Perel, S. (1991). Therapeutic factors in occupational therapy. *American Journal of Occupational Therapy, 45*, 59–66.

Ferencik, B. M. (1992). The helping process in group therapy: A review and discussion. *Group, 16*, 113–124.

Fidler, G. S. (1993). The quest for efficacy. *American Journal of Occupational Therapy, 47*, 583–586.

Finlay, L. (1993). *Groupwork in occupational therapy*. London: Chapman & Hall.

Flapan, D., & Fenchel, G. H. (1987). Terminations. *Group, 11*, 131–143.

Fleming, M. H. (1991). The therapist with the three-track mind. *American Journal of Occupational Therapy, 45*, 1007–1014.

Foy, J. (1994, May 9). Gender issues in the workplace. *The London Free Press*, p. B17

Frank, M. G. (1990). The use of self in group psychotherapy. *Group, 14*, 145–150.

Frank, J. D. (1992). Some determinants, manifestations, and effects of cohesiveness in therapy groups. In K. R. MacKenzie (Ed.), *Classics in group psychotherapy*. New York: Guilford.

Fridinger, F., Goodwin, G., & Chng, C. L. (1992). Physician and consumer attitudes and behaviors regarding self-help support groups as an adjunct to traditional medical care. *Journal of Health & Social Policy, 3*, 19–36.

Fried, E. (1972). Basic concepts in group psychotherapy. In H. I. Kaplan & B. J. Sadock (Eds.), *The evolution of group therapy* (pp. 27–50). New York: E. P. Dutton.

Funk and Wagnalls Standard College Dictionary (Cdn. ed.). (1982). Toronto: Fitzhenry & Whiteside.

Gabriel, M. A. (1993). The cotherapy relationship: Special issues and problems in AIDS therapy groups. *Group, 17*, 33–42.

Garland, J. A. (1992). Developing and sustaining group work services: A systemic and systematic view. *Social Work with Groups, 15*, 89–98.

Garvin, C. (1992). A task-centered group approach to work with the chronically mentally ill. *Social Work with Groups, 15*, 67–80.

Geller, L. (1982). The failure of self-actualization theory: A critique of Carl Rogers and Abraham Maslow. *Journal of Humanistic Psychology, 22*, 56–73.

Gemmill, G. (1986). The mythology of the leader role in small groups. *Small Group Behavior, 17*, 41–50.

Gersick, C. J. G. (1988). Time and transition in work terms: Toward a new model of group development. *Academy of Management Journal, 31*, 9–41.

Gibb, J. R., & Gibb L. M. (1978). The group as a growing organism. In L. P. Bradford (Ed.), *Group development* (pp. 104–116). La Jolla, CA: University Associates.

Gillette, J., & McCollom, M. (Eds.). (1990). *Groups in context*. Reading, MA: Addison-Wesley.

Ginsberg, C. (1984). Toward a more somatic understanding of self. *Journal of Humanistic Psychology, 24*, 66–92.

Gladding, S. T. (1991). *Group work: A counseling specialty*. New York: Macmillan.

Goldklang, D. S. (1991). Research workshop on methodological issues in evaluating preventive interventions using mutual support. *American Journal of Community Psychology, 19*, 789–795.

Goldman, M. (1965). A comparison of individual and group performance for varying combinations of initial ability. *Journal of Personality and Social Psychology, 1,* 210–216.

Goldstein, A. P., & Myers, C. R. (1986). Relationship enhancement methods. In F. H. Kanfer & A. P. Goldstein (Eds.), *Helping people change: A textbook of methods* (3d ed.) (pp. 19–65). New York: Pergamon Press

Gottlieb, B. H., & Peters, L. (1991). A national demographic portrait of mutual aid group participants in Canada. *American Journal of Community Psychology, 19,* 651–667.

Grady, A. P. (1994, July). *Building inclusive communities: A challenge for occupational therapy.* Eleanor Clarke Slagle lecture presented at the CAN-AM conference, Boston.

Greeley, A. T., Garcia, V. I., Kessler, B. L., & Gilchrest, G. (1992). Training effective multicultural group counselors: Issues for a group training course. *Journal for Specialists in Group Work, 17,* 196–209.

Green, M. C. (1994). Editorial. *National, 11,* 3.

Haaga, D. A., & Davison, G. C. (1986). Cognitive change methods. In F. H. Kanfer & A. P. Goldstein (Eds.), *Helping people change: A textbook of methods* (3d ed.) (pp. 236–282). New York: Pergamon.

Hall, A. D., & Fagen, R. E. (1968). Definition of a system. In W. Buckley (Ed.), *Modern system's research for the behavioural scientist* (pp. 81–92). Chicago: Aldine.

Halperin, D. (1987). The self-help group: The mental health professional's role. *Group, 11,* 47–53.

Handelsman, M. M., and Snyder, C. R. (1982). Is "rejected" feedback really rejected?: Effects of informativeness on reactions to positive and negative personality feedback. *Journal of Personality, 50,* 168–179.

Hansen, J. C., Warner, R. W., & Smith, E. M. (1980). *Group counseling: Theory and process* (2d ed.). Chicago: Rand McNally.

Hare, A. P. (1976). *Handbook of small group research* (2d ed.). New York: The Free Press.

Hare, A. P. (1992). *Groups, teams, and social interaction: Theories and applications.* New York: Praeger.

Heap, K. (1977). *Group theory for social workers.* Oxford: Pergammon Press.

Henry, A. D., Nelson, D. L., & Duncombe, L. W. (1984). Choice making in group and individual activity. *American Journal of Occupational Therapy, 38,* 245–251.

Heron, J. (1989). *The facilitator's handbook.* London: Kogan Page.

Howe, M. C. (1986). An occupational therapy activity group. *American Journal of Occupational Therapy, 22,* 176–179.

Howe, M. C., & Schwartzberg, S. L. (1986). *A functional approach to group work in occupational therapy.* Philadelphia: J. B. Lippincott.

Jacobs, E. E., Harvill, R. L., & Masson, R. L. (1988). *Group counseling: Strategies and skills.* Pacific Grove, CA: Brooks/Cole.

Jacobs, M. K, & Goodman, G. (1989). Psychology and self-help groups. *American Psychologist, 44,* 536–545.

Janov, A. (1972). *The primal revolution.* New York: Simon & Schuster.

Johnson, B. D. (1994, January 31). The male myth. *Macleans,* pp. 39–42.

Johnson, D. W., & Johnson, F. P. (1987). *Joining together: Group therapy and group skills* (3d ed.). Englewood Cliffs, NJ: Prentice-Hall.

Johnson, N P., & Phelps, G. L. (1991). Effectiveness in self-help groups: Alcoholics Anonymous as a prototype. *Community Health, 14*, 22–27.

Kanfer, F. H., & Goldstein, A. P. (1986). *Helping people change: A textbook of methods.* Elmsford, NY: Pergamon Press.

Kaplan, K. L. (1988). The directive group: Treatment for psychiatric patients with a minimum level of functioning. *American Journal of Occupational Therapy, 40*, 474–481.

Kassel, J. D., & Wagner, E. F. (1993). Processes of change in Alcoholics Anonymous: A review of possible mechanisms. *Psychotherapy, 30*, 223–234.

Katz, A., & Bender, E. I. (1976). Self-help groups in western society: History and prospects. *Journal of Applied Behavioral Science, 12*, 265–282.

Kees, N. L., & Jacobs, E. (1990). Conducting more effective groups: How to select and process group exercises. *Journal for Specialists in Group Work, 15*, 21–29.

Kenny, D. A., & De Paulo, B. M. (1993). Do people know how others view them? An empirical and theoretical account. *Psychological Bulletin, 114*, 145–161.

Kertay, L., & Reviere, S. L. (1993). The use of touch in psychotherapy: Theoretical and ethical considerations. *Psychotherapy, 30*, 32–40.

Keyton, J. (1993). Group termination: Completing the study of group development. *Small Group Research, 24*, 84–100,

King II, T. I. (1992). Hand strengthening with a computer for purposeful activity. *American Journal of Occupational Therapy, 47*, 635–637.

Kirchmeyer, C. (1993). Multicultural task groups. *Small Group Research, 24*, 127–148.

Kivlighan, D. M., & Angelone, E. O. (1992). Interpersonal problems: Variables influencing participants' perception of group climate. *Journal of Counseling Psychology, 39*, 468–472.

Kleinberg, J. L. (1991). Teaching beginning group therapists to incorporate a patient's empathic capacity in treatment planning. *Group, 15*, 141–151.

Korda, L. S., & Pancrazio, J. J. (1989). Limiting negative outcome in group practice. *Journal for Specialists in Group Work, 14*, 112–120.

Kottler, J. A. (1983). *Pragmatic group leadership.* Monterey, CA: Brooks/Cole.

Kremer, E. R. H., Nelson, D. L., & Duncombe, L. W. (1984). Effects of selected activities on affective meaning in psychiatric patients. *American Journal of Occupational Therapy, 38*, 522–528.

Kreps, G. L., & Thornton, B. C. (1984). *Health communication theory and practice.* New York: Longman.

Krupnick, J. L., Rowland, J. H., Golberg, R. L., & Daniel, U. V. (1993). Professionally led support groups for cancer patients: An intervention in search of a model. *International Journal of Psychiatry in Medicine, 23*, 275–294.

Kurtz, L. F. (1992). Group environment in self-help groups for families. *Small Group Research, 23*, 199–215.

Kurtz, L. F., & Powell, T. J. (1987). Three approaches to understanding self-help groups. *Social Work with Groups, 10*, 69–80.

Lacoursiere, R. (1980). *The life cycle of groups.* New York: Human Sciences Press.

LaFarge, V. V. S. (1990). Termination in groups. In J. Gillette & M. McCollom (Eds.), *Groups in context* (pp. 171–185). Reading, MA: Addison-Wesley.

Lakin, M. (1983). Experiential helping groups. In H. H. Blumberg, A. P. Hare, V. Kent, & M. Davies (Eds.), *Groups and social interaction* (pp. 209–226). New York: John Wiley & Sons.

Latham, Van M. (1987). Task type and group motivation. *Small Group Behavior, 18,* 56–71.

Lazarus, A. A. (1989). Multimodel therapy. In R. J. Corsini & D. Wedding (Eds.), *Current psychotherapies* (4th ed.) (pp. 503–544). Itasca, IL: F. E. Peacock

Levine, B. (1979). *Group psychotherapy: Practice and development.* Englewood Cliffs, NJ: Prentice-Hall.

Levine, R. E. (1987). The influence of the arts-and-crafts movement on the professional status of occupational therapy. *American Journal of Occupational Therapy, 41,* 248–254.

Levy, L. H. (1979). Processes and activities in groups. In M. A. Lieberman & L. D. Borman, *Self-help groups for coping with crisis* (pp. 234–271). San Francisco: Jossey-Bass.

Lewin, K., Lippitt, R., & White, R. K. (1939). Patterns of aggressive behavior in experimentally created "social climates." *Journal of Social Psychology, 10,* 271–299.

Lewis, P. (1987). Therapeutic change in groups: An interactional perspective. *Small Group Behavior, 18,* 548–556.

Lieberman, M. A. (1979). Analyzing change mechanisms in groups. In M. A. Lieberman & L. D. Borman, *Self-help groups for coping with crisis* (pp. 194–233). San Francisco: Jossey-Bass.

Lieberman, M. A. (1983). Comparative analyses of change mechanisms in groups. In H. H. Blumberg, A. P. Hare, & M. Davies (Eds.), *Small groups and social interaction* (pp. 239–252). New York: John Wiley & Sons.

Lieberman, M. A. (1990a). A group therapist perspective on self-help groups. *International Journal of Group Psychotherapy, 40,* 251–278.

Lieberman, M. A. (1990b). Understanding how groups work: A study of homogeneous peer group failures. *International Journal of Group Psychotherapy, 40,* 31–52.

Lieberman, M. A., & Borman, L. (1979). *Self-help groups for coping with crises.* San Francisco: Jossey-Bass.

Lieberman, M. A., & Videka-Sherman, L. (1986). The impact of self-help groups on the mental health of widows and widowers. *American Journal of Orthopsychiatry, 56,* 435–449.

Lieberman, M. A., Yalom, I. D., & Miles, M. B. (1973). *Encounter groups: First facts.* New York: Basic Books.

Llewelyn, S. P., & Haslett, A. V. J. (1986). Factors perceived as helpful by the members of self-help groups: An exploratory study. *British Journal of Guidance and Counselling, 14,* 252–262.

Long, L., & Cope, C. (1980). Curative factors in a male felony offender group. *Small Group Behavior, 11,* 389–398.

Luft, J. (1984). *Group processes, an introduction to group dynamics* (3d ed.). Palo Alto, CA: Mayfield.

MacDevitt, J. W., & Sanislow, C. (1987). Curative factors in offenders' groups. *Small Group Behavior, 18,* 72–81.

MacKenzie, K. R. (1987). Therapeutic factors in group psychotherapy: A contemporary view. *Group, 11,* 26–34.

MacKenzie, K. R., & Livesley, W. J. (1983). A developmental model for brief group therapy. In R. R. Dies & K. R. MacKenzie (Eds.), *Advances in group psychotherapy: Integrating research and practice* (pp. 101–116). New York: International Universities Press.

Madara, E. J. (1986). A comprehensive systems approach to promoting mutual aid self-help groups: The New Jersey self-help clearinghouse model. *Journal of Voluntary Action Research, 15,* 57–63.

Markowitz, M., & Kadis, A. L. (1972). Short-term analytic treatment of married couples in a group by a therapist couple. In C. J. Sager & H. S. Kaplan (Eds.), *Progress in group and family therapy.* New York: Brunner/Mazel.

Maslow, A. (1968). *Toward a psychology of being* (2d ed.). Princeton: Van Nostrand Reinhold.

Matthews, C. O. (1992). An application of general system theory (GST) to group therapy. *The Journal for Specialists in Group Work, 17,* 161–169.

Matthews, K. A., Batson, C. D., Horn, J., & Rosenman, R. H. (1981). "Principles in his nature which interest him in the fortune of others . . .": The heritability of empathic concern for others. *Journal of Personality, 49,* 237–247.

Mattingly, C. (1991). What is clinical reasoning? *American Journal of Occupational Therapy, 45,* 979–986.

McCollom, M. (1990). Group formation: Boundaries, leadership, and culture. In J. Gillette & M. McCollom (Eds.), *Groups in context* (pp. 34–48). Reading, MA: Addison-Wesley.

McLees, E., Margo, G. M., Waterman, S., & Beeber, A. (1992). Group climate and group development in a community meeting on a short-term inpatient psychiatric unit. *Group, 16,* 18–30.

McNary, S. W., & Dies, R. R. (1993). Cotherapist modeling in group psychotherapy: Fact or fantasy. *Group, 17,* 131–142.

Meissen, G. J., Mason, W. C., & Gleason, D. F. (1991). Understanding the attitudes and intentions of future professionals toward self-help. *American Journal of Community Psychology, 19,* 699–714)

Miller, L., & Nelson, D. L. (1987). Dual-purpose activity versus single-purpose activity in terms of duration on task, exertion level, and affect. *Occupational Therapy in Mental Health, 7,* 55–67.

Mitchell, T. R., & Silver, W. S. (1990). Individual and group goals when workers are interdependent: Effects on task strategies and performance. *Journal of Applied Psychology, 75,* 185–193.

Moos, R. (1986). *Group environment scale manual* (2d ed.). Palo Alto, CA: Consulting Psychologists Press.

Moreno, J. L. (1957). *The first book on group psychotherapy.* New York: Beacon House.

Moreno, J. L. (1977). *Psychodrama: First volume* (4th ed.). New York: Beacon House.

Morganett, R. S. (1990). *Skills for living: Group counseling activities for young adolescents.* Champaign, IL: Research Press.

Mosey, A. C. (1986). *Psychosocial components of occupational therapy.* New York: Raven Press.

Mullen, H. (1992). "Existential" therapists and their group therapy practices. *International Journal of Group Psychotherapy, 42,* 453–468.

Napier, R. W., & Gershenfeld, M. K. (1989). *Groups: Theory and experience* (4th ed.). Boston: Houghton Mifflin.

Natiello, P. (1987). The person-centered approach: From theory to practice. *Person-Centered Review, 2*, 203–216.

Nelson, A., Mackenthun, D., Bloesch, A., Milan, A., Unrein, M., & Hill, K. (1956). A preliminary report on a study in group occupational therapy. *American Journal of Occupational Therapy, 10*, 254–258, 262–263, 271.

Nelson, D. L., Peterson, C., Smith, D. A., Boughton, J. A., & Whalen, G. M. (1988). Effects of project versus parallel groups on social interaction and affective responses in senior citizens. *American Journal of Occupational Therapy, 42*, 23–29.

Nelson-Jones, R. (1990b). *Human relationships: A skills approach*. Pacific Grove, CA: Brooks/Cole.

Nelson-Jones, R. (1992). *Group leadership: A training approach*. Pacific Grove, CA: Brooks/Cole.

New Lexicon Webster's Dictionary, The (1987). New York: Lexicon Publications.

Orme, M. E. J. (1987). Uses of humour in instruction. *Reflections, 25*, 1–4.

Ormont, L. R. (1992). *The group therapy experience*. New York: St. Martin's Press.

Paine, A. L., Suarez-Balcazar, Y., Fawcett, S.B., & Borck-Jameson, L. (1992). Supportive transactions: Their measurement and enhancement in two mutual-aid groups. *Journal of Community Psychology, 20*, 163–180.

Palazzolo, C. S. (1981). *Small groups: An introduction*. New York: Van Nostrand Reinhold.

Pellegrini, R. J. (1971). Some effects of seating position on social perception. *Psychological Reports, 28*, 887–893.

Peloquin, S. M. (1993). The Depersonalization of Patients: A profile gleaned from narratives. *American Journal of Occupational Therapy, 47*, 830–837.

Peloquin, S. M. (1994). Moral treatment: How a caring practice lost its rationale. *American Journal of Occupational Therapy, 48*, 167–173.

Perkins, V. J. (1992). A model for selecting leadership styles. *Occupational Therapy in Health Care, 8*, 225–237.

Pollak, G. K. (1975). *Leadership of discussion groups*. New York: Spectrum.

Posthuma, A. B., & Posthuma, B. W. (1973). Some observations on encounter group casualties. *Journal of Applied Behavioural Science, 9*, 595–608.

Posthuma, B. W. (1972). Personal development and occupational therapy. *American Journal of Occupational Therapy, 26*, 88–90.

Posthuma, B. W. (1976). A deprivation experience. *Canadian Journal of Occupational Therapy, 43*, 129–130.

Posthuma, B. W. (1985). Learning to touch. *Canadian Journal of Occupational Therapy, 52*, 189–193.

Posthuma, B. W., & Posthuma, A. B. (1972). The effect of a small-group experience on occupational therapy students. *American Journal of Occupational Therapy, 26*, 415–418.

Powell, T. J. (1987). *Self-help organizations and professional practice*. Silver Spring, MD: National Association of Social Workers.

Powell, T. J. (1990). *Working with self-help*. Silver Spring, MD: National Association of Social Workers.

Powell, T. J., & Cameron, M. J. (1991). Self-help research and the public mental health system. *American Journal of Community Psychology, 19*, 797–805.

Prazoff, M., Joyce, A. S., & Azim, H. F. A. (1986). Brief crises group psychotherapy: One therapist's model. *Group, 10*, 34–40.

Punwar, A. J. (1994). *Occupational therapy: Principles and practice* (2d ed.). Baltimore: Williams & Wilkins.

Purtilo, R. (1978). *Health professional/patient interaction*. Philadelphia: W. B. Saunders.

Rachman, A. W. (1990). Judicious self-disclosure in group analysis. *Group, 14*, 132–144.

Ramey, J. H. (1992). Group work practice in neighborhood centers to-day. *Social Work with Groups, 15*, 193–206.

Ramsey, P. W. (1992). Characteristics, processes, and effectiveness of community support groups: A review of the literature. *Family and Community Health, 15*, 38–48.

Rapoport, A. (1968). Forward. In W. Buckley (Ed.), *Modern systems research for the behavioral scientist* (pp. xiii–xxii). Chicago: Aldine.

Raskin, N. J., & Rogers, C. R. (1989). Person-centered therapy. In R. J. Corsini & D. Wedding (Eds.), *Current psychotherapies* (4th ed.) (pp. 155–194). Itasca, IL: F. E. Peacock.

Revenson, T. A., & Cassel, J. B. (1991). An exploration of leadership in a medical mutual help organization. *American Journal of Community Psychology, 19*, 683–698.

Roberts, L. J., Luke, D. A., Rappaport, J., Seidman, E., Toro, P. A., & Reischl, T. M. (1991). Charting uncharted terrain: A behavioral observation system for mutual help groups. *American Journal of Community Psychology, 19*, 715–737.

Rogers, C. R. (1951). *Client-centered therapy*. Boston: Houghton Mifflin.

Rogers, C. R. (1961). *On becoming a person*. Boston: Houghton Mifflin.

Rogers, C. R. (1985). Comment on Slack's article. *Journal of Humanistic Psychology, 25*, 43–44.

Romeder, J. M. (1990). *The self-help way: Mutual aid and health*. Ottawa, Ont., Canada: Canadian Council on Social Development.

Rootes, L. E., & Aanes, D. L. (1992). A conceptual framework for understanding self-help groups. *Hospital and Community Psychiatry, 43*, 379–381.

Rose, S. D. (1986). Co-therapy. In M. Rosenbaum & M. Berger (Eds.). *Group psychotherapy and group function* (Rev. ed.) (pp. 389–408). New York: Basic Books.

Rosenbaum, M. (1976). Group psychotherapy. In M. Rosenbaum & A. Snadowsky (Eds.), *The intensive group experience* (pp. 1–49). New York: Free Press.

Rosenbaum, M., & Berger, M. M. (1975). *Group psychotherapy and group function* (Rev. ed.). New York: Basic Books.

Ross, M. (1991). *Integrative group therapy*. Thorofare, NJ: Slack.

Rudestam, K. E. (1982). *Experiential groups in theory and practice*. Monterey, CA: Brooks/Cole.

Rugel, R. P. (1991). Closed and open systems: The Tavistock group from a general system perspective. *Journal for Specialists in Group Work, 16*, 74–84.

Saavedra, R., Earley, P. C., & Van Dyne, L. (1993). Complex interdependence in task-performing groups. *Journal of Applied Psychology, 78*, 61–72.

Sadock, B. J., & Kaplan, H. I. (1972). Selection of patients and the dynamic and structural organization of the group. In H. I. Kaplan & B. J. Sadock (Eds.), *The evolution of group therapy* (pp. 119–131). New York: E. P. Dutton.

Saint-Jean, M., & Desrosiers, L. (1993). Psychoanalytic considerations regarding the occupational therapy setting for treatment of the psychotic patient. *Occupational*

Therapy in Mental Health, 12, 69–78.

Sampson, E. E., & Marthas, M. (1981). *Group process for the health professions* (2d ed.). New York: Wiley.

Scheidlinger, S., & Schamess, G. (1992). Fifty years of AGPA 1942–1992: An overview. In K. R. Mackenzie (Ed.), *Classics in group psychotherapy* (pp. 1–22). New York: Guilford Press.

Schell. B. A., & Cervero, R. M. (1993). Clinical reasoning in occupational therapy: An integrative review. *American Journal of Occupational Therapy, 47,* 605–610.

Schroeder, H. M., & Harvey, O. J. (1963). Conceptual organization and group structure. In O. J. Harvey (Ed.), *Motivation and social interaction* (pp. 134–166). New York: Ronald Press.

Schubert, M. A., & Borkman, T. J. (1991). An organizational typology for self-help groups. *American Journal of Community Psycholgy, 19,* 769–787.

Schultz, B. (1986). Communication correlates of perceived leaders in the small group. *Small Group Behavior, 17,* 51–65.

Schulz, C. H. (1993). Helping factors in a peer-developed support group for persons with head injury, Part 2: Survivor interview perspective. *American Journal of Occupational Therapy, 48,* 305–309.

Schwartzben, S. H. (1992). Social work with multi-family groups: A partnership model for long-term care settings. *Social Work in Health Care, 18,* 23–38.

Schwartzberg, S. L. (1993). Helping factors in a peer-developed support group for persons with head injury, Part 1: Participant observer perspective. *American Journal of Occupational Therapy, 48,* 297–304.

Seashore, C. (1974). Time and transition in the intensive group experience. In A. Jacobs & W. W. Spradlin (Eds.), *The group as agent of change.* New York: Behavioral Publications.

Shaffer, J. B., & Galinsky, M. D. (1989). *Models of group therapy* (2d ed.). Englewood Cliffs, NJ: Prentice-Hall.

Shannon, P. D., & Snortum, J. R. (1965). An activity group's role. *American Journal of Occupational Therapy, XIX,* 344–347.

Shapiro, J. L. (1978). *Methods of group psychotherapy: A tradition of innovation.* Itasca, IL: F. E. Peacock.

Sherman, S. J., & Fazio, R. H. (1983). Parallels between attitudes and traits as predictors of behavior. *Journal of Personality, 51,* 308–345.

Shoemaker, G. (1987). A study of human relations training groups: Leadership style and outcome. *Small Group Behavior, 18,* 356–366.

Sklare, G., Keener, R., & Mas, C. (1990). Preparing members for "here-and-now" group counseling. *Journal for Specialists in Group Work, 15,* 141–148.

Slavin, R. L. (1993). The significance of here-and-now disclosure in promoting cohesion in group psychotherapy. *Group, 17,* 143–149.

Slavson, S. R. (1992). Are there group dynamics in therapy groups? In K. R. MacKenzie (Ed.), *Classics in group psychotherapy* (pp. 166–182). New York: Guilford Press.

Smith, K. K. (1990). On using the self as instrument: Lessons from a facilitator's experience. In J. Gillette & M. McCollom (Eds.), *Groups in context* (pp. 276–294). Reading, MA: Addison-Wesley.

Smith, P. B. (1980a). *Group processes and personal change.* London: Harper &

Row.

Smith, P. B. (Ed.). (1980b). *Small groups and personal change*. London: Methuen.

Smith, P. B., Wood, H., & Smale, G. G. (1980). The usefulness of groups in clinical settings. In P. B. Smith (Ed.), *Small groups and personal change*. New York: Methuen.

Snyder, C. R., Ingram, R. E., Handelsman, M. M., & Wells, D. S. (1982). Desire for personal feedback: Who wants it and what does it mean for psychotherapy? *Journal of Personality*, *50*, 316–330.

Srivastva, S., & Barrett, F. J. (1988). The transforming nature of metaphors in group development: A study in group theory. *Human Relations*, *41*, 31–64.

Stake, J. E. (1983). Situation and person-centered approaches to promoting leadership behavior in low-performance self-esteem women. *Journal of Personality*, *51*, 62–77.

Steffan, J. A. (1990). Productive occupation in small task groups of adults: Synthesis and annotations of the social psychology literature. In American Occupational Therapy Association, *Reviews of selected literature on occupation and health* (pp. 175–281). Rockville, MD: American Occupational Therapy Association.

Steffan, L. A., & Nelson, D. L. (1987). The effects of tool scarcity on group climate and affective meaning within the context of a stenciling activity. *American Journal of Occupational Therapy*, *41*, 449–453.

Steinbeck, T. M. (1986). Purposeful activity and performance. *American Journal of Occupational Therapy*, *40*, 529–534.

Stempler, B. L. (1993). Supervisory co-leadership: An innovative model for teaching the use of social group work in clinical social work training. *Social Work with Groups*, *16*, 97–110.

Stewart, M. J. (1990). Professional interface with mutual-aid self-help groups: A review. *Social Science Medicine*, *31*, 1143–1158.

Stockton, R., Rohde, R. I., & Haughey, J. (1992). The effects of structured group exercises on cohesion, engagement, avoidance, and conflict. *Small Group Research*, *23*, 155–168.

Stogdill, R. M. (1969). Personal factors associated with leadership: A survey of the literature. In C. A. Gibb (Ed.), *Leadership* (pp. 91–133). Harmondsworth, England: Penguin Books.

Svidén, G., & Säljö, R. (1993). Perceiving patients and their nonverbal reactions. *American Journal of Occupational Therapy*, *47*, 491–497.

Tannen, D. (1990). *You just don't understand*. New York: Ballantine Books.

Tannenbaum, R., & Schmidt, W. H. (1958). How to choose a leadership pattern. *Harvard Business Review*, *36*, 95–101.

Tebes, J. K., & Kraemer, D. T. (1991). Quantitative and qualitative knowing in mutual support research: Some lessons from the recent history of scientific psychology. *American Journal of Community Psychology*, *19*, 739–756.

Tollerud, T. R., Holling, D. W., & Dustin, D. (1992). A model for teaching in group leadership: The pre-group interview application. *Journal for Specialists in Group Work*, *17*, 96–104.

Tooper, V. O. (1984). Humor as an adjunct to occupational therapy interactions. *Occupational Therapy in Health Care*, *1*, 49–59.

Toothman, J. M. (1978). *Conducting the small group experience*. Washington: University Press of America.

Trojan, A. (1989). Benefits of self-help groups: A survey of 232 members from 65 disease-related groups. *Social Science Medicine, 29,* 225–232.

Trotzer, J. P. (1977). *The counselor and the group: Integrating theory, training, and practice.* Monterey, CA: Brooks/Cole.

Tuckman, B. W. (1965). Developmental sequence in small groups. *Psychological Bulletin, 63,* 384–399.

Tuckman, B. W., & Jensen, M. A. C. (1977). Stages of small group development revisited. *Group and Organization Studies, 2,* 419–427.

Tyson, T. (1989). *Working with groups.* Melbourne, Australia: Macmillan.

Tziner, A., & Eden, D. (1985). Effects of crew composition on crew performance: Does the whole equal the sum of its parts? *Journal of Applied Psychology, 70,* 85–93.

Urbanowski, R., & Vargo, J. (1994). Spirituality, daily practice, and the occupational performance model. *Canadian Journal of Occupational Therapy, 61,* 88–94.

Vacc, N. A. (1989). Group counseling: C. H. Patterson—A personalized view. *Journal for Specialists in Group Work, 14,* 4–15.

Verba, S. (1961). *Small groups and political behavior: A study of leadership.* Princeton: Princeton University Press.

Verdi, A. F., & Wheelan, S. A. (1992). Developmental patterns in same-sex and mixed-sex groups. *Small Group Research, 23,* 356–378.

Vergeer, G., & MacRae, A. (1993). Therapeutic use of humor in occupational therapy. *American Journal of Occupational Therapy, 47,* 678–683.

Waldinger, R. J. (1990). *Psychiatry for medical students* (2d ed.). Washington, DC: American Psychiatric Press.

Webster, D., & Schwartzberg, S. L. (1992). Patients' perception of curative factors in occupational therapy groups. *Occupational Therapy in Mental Health, 12,* 3–24.

Wells, L. (1990). The group as a whole: A systematic socioanalytic perspective on interpersonal and group relations. In J. Gillette & M. McCollom (Eds.), *Groups in context* (pp. 49–85). Reading, MA: Addison-Wesley.

Wheelan, S. A., & McKeage, R. L. (1993). Developmental patterns in small and large groups. *Small Group Research, 24,* 60–83.

Wolf, A. (1975). Psychoanalysis in groups. In M. Rosenbaum & M. M. Berger (Eds.), *Group psychotherapy and group function* (Rev. ed.) (pp. 321–335). New York: Basic Books.

Wollert, R. (1987a). Human services and the self-help clearinghouse concept. *Canadian Journal of Community Mental Health, 6,* 79–90.

Wollert, R., & The Self-Help Research Team. (1987b). The self-help clearinghouse concept: An evaluation of one program and its implications for policy and practice. *American Journal of Community Psychology, 15,* 491–508.

Yalom, I. D. (1983). *Inpatient group psychotherapy.* New York: Basic Books.

Yalom, I. D. (1985). *Theory and practice of group psychotherapy* (3d ed.). New York: Basic Books.

YWCA of Metropolitan Toronto. (1991). *Discovering life skills* (Vol. VI). Toronto, Ont., Canada: Author.

Appendices

Appendices A and B contain examples of how to plan and organize a series of group sessions around the central themes of assertiveness and awareness, respectively. Suggested activities and exercises for six sessions on each theme are included. Depending on the functional level of the members, the content presented may be appropriate as laid out for six sessions or it may need to be reorganized into additional or fewer sessions.

Recommendations are included as to the types of problems that can be addressed in the sessions. There are some minimal functional requirements that clients must meet in order to benefit from the sessions as they are laid out, and these limitations are included as recommendations for client selection.

The format used here has the general objectives for the overall experience (six sessions) presented at the beginning. In a similar way the leader will want to formulate specific objectives for each session relative to the needs of group members.

APPENDIX A

Small Group Program

Theme: Assertiveness

Sessions: Six

Recommendations:

For these problem areas:

1. Anxiety
2. Difficulty speaking spontaneously
3. Low self-esteem
4. Low self-confidence
5. Nonassertive approach to others
6. Aggressive approach to others

For clients who are:

1. Functionally literate
2. Able to interact verbally at least at a minimal level
3. Cognitively alert

Objectives:

1. To improve awareness, recognition, and expression of feelings in an appropriate manner, both verbally and nonverbally
2. To enable differentiation between assertive, nonassertive, and aggressive behavior
3. To practice assertive rights and responsibilities in order to increase self-respect and self-esteem as well as to gain respect from others
4. To learn basic conversational skills in order to reduce social anxieties
5. To learn appropriate ways of making and refusing requests
6. To learn a problem-solving approach to clearer communication through familiarization of the DESC system (i.e., format for an assertive response)
7. To learn coping skills in dealing with manipulation and unfair criticism

Effective Aids:

1. Structured exercises
2. Suggested situations for role plays
3. Printed handouts or manuals
4. Posters
5. Flip chart or blackboard
6. Homework assignments

Topics:

Session 1: Nonassertive behaviors; aggressive behaviors
Session 2: Assertive behaviors; nonverbal components of behaviors
Session 3: Barriers to being assertive; the ABC of emotions
Session 4: Assertiveness rights and responsibilities; principles of assertiveness; the DESC script
Session 5: Broken record; workable compromise
Session 6: Building self-respect; coping with criticism

SESSION 1

Nonassertive Behavior

The aim of nonassertive behaviors is to please others and to *avoid conflict* at any cost. It results in the loss of self-respect. When you are nonassertive, what message are you actually conveying to others? (Try to get group members to offer ideas similar to the ones that follow.)

Nonassertive behavior says, in effect:

"You're O.K, I'm not O.K."

"I don't count."

"My feelings don't matter."

"I don't respect myself."

Exercise 1   This exercise will help you recognize how often you behave in the following nonassertive ways:

	Always	*Often*	*Sometimes*	*Never*
1. Letting others take the initiative in starting conversations	_____	_____	_____	_____
2. Being unable to refuse requests for your time, energy, or money	_____	_____	_____	_____
3. Failing to express your feelings or opinions when you would like to do so	_____	_____	_____	_____
4. Not accepting a compliment when you would like to do so	_____	_____	_____	_____
5. Being unable to give a compliment when you would like to do so	_____	_____	_____	_____

	Always	Often	Sometimes	Never
6. Letting criticism over-whelm you without saying anything	_____	_____	_____	_____
7. Having difficulty giving criticism or giving a compliment	_____	_____	_____	_____
8. Frequently apologizing for or justifying your behavior to others	_____	_____	_____	_____

Discussion by members about their answers to the examples should follow. Figure A–1 exemplifies that nonassertive behavior invites others to "walk over us."

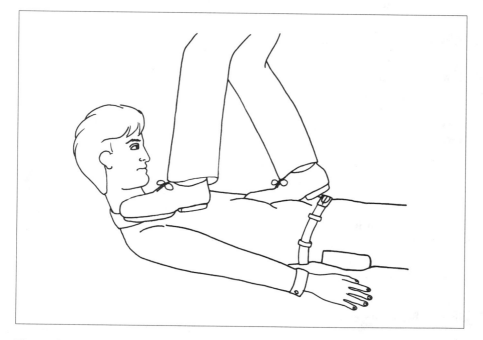

Figure A–1.   Nonassertive behavior invites being walked over.

Aggressive Behavior

The aim of aggressive behavior is to achieve or maintain control over people or situations. It can cause others to feel humiliated, put down, and angry. When you are being aggressive, what message are you really sending to others? (Try to get members to offer ideas similar to the ones that follow.)

Aggressive behavior says in effect:

"I'm O.K., you're not O.K."

"This is what I want, think, or feel. You have no right to want, think, or feel otherwise".

"You don't count."

"I don't respect you."

Exercise 2   Below is a list of some of the ways people behave aggressively. Read the list and in the columns at the right, indicate how frequently you behave aggressively in these ways.

	Always	*Often*	*Sometimes*	*Never*
1. Speaking for others	_____	_____	_____	_____
2. Making judgments on who or what is right or wrong; telling another person what he or she should or should not do	_____	_____	_____	_____
3. Commanding, persuading, directing, controlling, manipulating other people in *personal* situations	_____	_____	_____	_____
4. Insulting or putting down others	_____	_____	_____	_____
5. Belittling others or calling them names	_____	_____	_____	_____
6. Being so rude you destroy relationships	_____	_____	_____	_____
7. Making insulting gestures, signs, or faces	_____	_____	_____	_____

Share and discuss responses.

Exercise 3   Complete the following with (1) an aggressive response, and (2) a nonassertive response:

An acquaintance has asked to borrow your car for the evening but you have planned to use it. You say:

1. _____

_____

_____

2. _____

_____

_____

Group members share their responses and discuss them.

SESSION 2

Assertive Behaviors

The aim of assertive behaviors is to leave us feeling satisfied with our interactions. It allows us to express our thoughts, feelings, and beliefs in a manner that does not violate the rights of others. When you are being assertive, what message are you conveying to others? (Try to facilitate members' offering ideas similar to the ones that follow.)

Assertive behavior says, in effect:

"I'm, O.K., you're O.K."

"I respect both myself and you."

"I expect you to respect me."

Exercise 4   Assertiveness does not mean simply being able to say "no." Learn to recognize your assertive behavior. Indicate in the columns at the right how often you behave assertively in doing the following:

	Always	*Often*	*Sometimes*	*Never*
1. Saying I like, I prefer, my opinion is, I feel . . .	_____	_____	_____	_____
2. Telling others about your abilities, interests	_____	_____	_____	_____
3. Carrying on a conversation	_____	_____	_____	_____
4. Giving and receiving	_____	_____	_____	_____
5. Making your actions (nonverbal behavior) match your words	_____	_____	_____	_____
6. Disagreeing with others	_____	_____	_____	_____
7. Asking for directions, reasons, or to have something made clear	_____	_____	_____	_____
8. Being persistent in making requests, in disagreeing, or in standing your ground	_____	_____	_____	_____

	Always	Often	Sometimes	Never
9. Coping with criticism in a reasonably comfortable manner	_____	_____	_____	_____
10. Speaking without excusing, justifying, or apologizing for yourself	_____	_____	_____	_____
11. Knowing your rights and responsibilities and respecting them	_____	_____	_____	_____
12. Being in control of yourself and your behavior, feelings, and thoughts	_____	_____	_____	_____
13. Looking and feeling confident about yourself	_____	_____	_____	_____

Exercise 5 Complete the following example with an assertive response: You are expecting an important telephone call before six o'clock. It is now five o'clock. Someone asks you to pick up a few items from the convenience store before it closes at six o'clock.

You say: _____

_____

_____

Share and discuss responses.

Nonverbal Components of Behaviors

Because the majority of our communication is carried out nonverbally (i.e., by what others see us do rather than by what we say), it is important to be aware of the kinds of messages we give, for example, through facial expressions and hand movements.

Exercise 6 In the following exercise, describe briefly the kind of nonverbal behavior that usually accompanies each of the three kinds of behavior listed across the top.

	Assertive	*Nonassertive*	*Aggressive*
Eye contact			
Body posture			
Hand movements			
Facial expression			

Note: This exercise can be done individually by handing out copies of it to each member (see example), or it can be done collectively by the members using a large chart drawn on a flip chart, blackboard, or poster. Either way, each member's contribution should be discussed by the group.

Exercise 6 Example

	Assertive	*Nonassertive*	*Aggressive*
Eye Contact	Direct	None	Staring
Body	Erect	Slumped	Forward
Hand movements	Natural	Tentative	Pronounced
Facial expression	Friendly	Downcast	Contorted

SESSION 3

Barriers to Being Assertive

Note: First, try to facilitate contributions by the group members to elicit the following five barriers and suggestions as to ways in which they affect individuals. The members can also be involved by having them write the barriers on a flip chart or blackboard.

1. *Anxiety.* We may not act assertively because of anxiety about what would happen as a result of our assertiveness. For example, we may fear hurting someone's feelings, being criticized, or even losing a friend.

2. *Guilt.* We may believe that we should always be able to please others. If we fail to do this, for example, by refusing a request, we may feel guilty. To avoid this feeling of guilt, we then may avoid acting assertively whenever we feel we might displease someone.

3. *Fear of feeling/looking ignorant or stupid.* We may avoid expressing our ideas assertiveley or asking questions because we are afraid of feeling or looking stupid.

4. *Irrational beliefs.* These beliefs, by definition, are not based on reality. They are beliefs which are not reasonable or sensible and make it difficult for us to be assertive. We develop irrational beliefs by focusing on the worst possible results and ignoring all the good possibilities of assertive behaviors. For example, "I should be perfect in everything I do." Such a belief stops one from taking chances or accepting one's mistakes. It is unrealistic to think that anyone can be perfect. To overcome these beliefs, we must challenge them and replace them with sensible, constructive ideas.

5. *Negative self-statements.* Negative self-statements are put-downs. Many of us continually put ourselves down. We say things to ourselves that are damaging to our self-respect and self-confidence (e.g., "I'm so stupid" . . . "I never do anything right"). Saying this kind of thing to ourselves and believing it keeps us from feeling good about ourselves. We are then reluctant to try new activities and miss opportunities to enjoy ourselves. It is important, therefore, to recognize our personal put-

downs and to challenge them. As we change the way we think, we will change the way we feel.

Exercise 7 The following are some commonly held irrational beliefs. Below each one, write a positive phrase to replace each italicized negative portion of the statement.

  a. If I say what I really think, *people won't like me.*

   If I say what I really think, _____

  b. If I refuse to do a favor for someone, *they will not be my friend any longer.*

   If I refuse to do a favor for someone, _____

In the space below, write a few of your own irrational beliefs and statements with which to challenge them.

_____

_____

_____

_____

Exercise 8 Write two of your personal put-downs. After each one, write a challenge or a correction of the put-down.

_____

_____

_____

_____

The ABC of Emotions

If we follow the A-B-C format outlined here we can change the way we think which will change the way we feel.

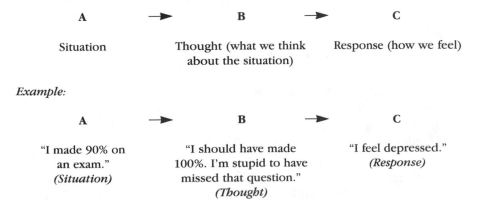

A	→	B	→	C
Situation		Thought (what we think about the situation)		Response (how we feel)

Example:

A	→	B	→	C
"I made 90% on an exam." *(Situation)*		"I should have made 100%. I'm stupid to have missed that question." *(Thought)*		"I feel depressed." *(Response)*

It is what we think or what we tell ourselves that causes us to feel depressed.

Exercise 9   Think of a situation and then think of a negative thought and response to that situation. Then, replace the negative thought and response with a positive thought and the response that follows.

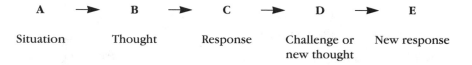

A	B	C	D	E
Situation	Thought	Response	Challenge or new thought	New response

We can challenge thoughts that leave us feeling put-down and develop new thoughts that help us to maintain our self-respect and self-confidence. Then, we will be able to accept ourselves and react to situations in a more relaxed, less stressful way.

SESSION 4

Assertiveness Rights and Responsibilities

The first step in learning to behave assertively is to become aware of, and eventually feel comfortable with, our assertiveness rights and their accompanying responsibilities.

Exercise 10   Here is a list of commonly accepted personal assertiveness rights. Read the list. Then in the column at the right, write the name of a person or situation where accepting this right would help you.

Right

A situation or person where this right would help you

1. I have the right to use my own judgment because I am responsible for myself

   _____

2. I have the right to be treated with respect

   _____

3. I have the right to have and express my own feelings

   _____

4. I have the right to be listened to and taken seriously

   _____

5. I have the right to set my own priorities

   _____

6. I have the right to say "no" without feeling guilty

   _____

Every right has one or more accompanying responsibilities. "I have the right to express my opinions"—the accompanying responsibility is to listen to and show respect for other people's right to express their opinions.

Exercise 11 For each right in the preceding list, write one or more accompanying responsibilities.

PRINCIPLES OF ASSERTIVENESS

1. Everyone has basic personal rights.
2. We cannot change others—only ourselves.
3. We are responsible for ourselves and our behaviors.
4. If we change our behaviors so that we feel more self-respect, people will respond differently to us.
5. No one can read minds successfully. We cannot know what others are thinking or feeling unless we ask them. Attempting to do so makes for poor communication.
6. We can *learn* to be assertive.

The DESC Script

A description of the DESC script follows. Use it to help plan or rehearse situations you find difficult to handle. It will help you to avoid saying things in a self-defeating or ineffective way. DESC is formed from the key words in the four steps: *D*escribe, *E*xpress, *S*pecify, and *C*onsequence.

Step 1: Describe. Describe to your partner the exact behaviors that are uncomfortable to you. Be as fair and clear as possible. Do not generalize or guess people's motives. You may start with sentences like, "I would like to discuss a matter with you" or "I've noticed that . . ."

Example: "As I understand it, you are asking me to drive to six hockey games again this year."

Step 2: Express. Say what you think and feel about the behaviors that bother you. Start your sentences with "I feel . . . ," "I believe . . . ," or "I think . . ." Avoid sarcasm and emotional outbursts. The goal is to let your partner know how her or his behaviors affect you.

Example: "I think that is more than my share of driving. It is very costly both in gasoline and my own time."

Step 3: Specify. The third step is to ask for different, clearly stated behaviors. Essentially you ask, "Please stop doing X and start doing Y instead." Best results occur when only one clearly stated request is made. Refer to changes in what your partner is *doing,* not to personality traits or attitudes. Be prepared for the other person to make requests for changes on your part.

Example: "Please change your list so that I am called on only three times during the year."

Step 4: Consequences. Emphasize the positive consequences that will follow if your request is met. Avoid threats or punishment if an agreement is not reached.

Example: "That way, I'll be glad to help with the driving."

Exercise 12   Use the DESC script to address the following examples:

   a. A friend often telephones you late at night to talk. There is no urgency to her calls and this evening she called you at 11:35 P.M., just to chat. You have to get up early in the morning for work and would prefer she call at an earlier time.

   b. You have been waiting in the supermarket line to check out your groceries. You are in a hurry and a man pushes his way in front of you saying he is in a rush and has only one item to check out.

Note: Other or additional scenarios that are appropriate for the particular members of your group might be used in place of, or in addition to, the two suggested here.

SESSION 5

Broken Record

Some people give up easily when they are opposed by others. In fact, most of us do in some situations. What we need to learn is to persist or to stick with it in saying where we stand in matters that are important to us. *Broken record* is a skill that helps us do this by repeating our position over and over without becoming rude or losing control of our behaviors.

The aim of using the broken record skill is to be persistent, as in Figure A–2, in holding a position in a disagreement or in making a request. The effect, after practice, is to enable you to become increasingly confident in expressing and holding your position.

Example:

   CHILD: Mom, may I watch TV now?

   PARENT: No, not until your homework is done.

   CHILD: But the cartoons are on!

   PARENT: I know you like to watch cartoons, but no, not until your homework is done.

   CHILD: You never let me watch what I want!

   PARENT: I know that you want to watch TV, but no, not until your homework is done.

Workable Compromise

Sometimes it is neither possible nor appropriate for us to get our own way and in most situations it is possible to reach a compromise. The key point in making a compromise is to make sure that the outcome does not lessen the self-respect of either person. This does not necessarily mean that each person gets an equal division of goods or choices, or an equal amount of satisfaction.

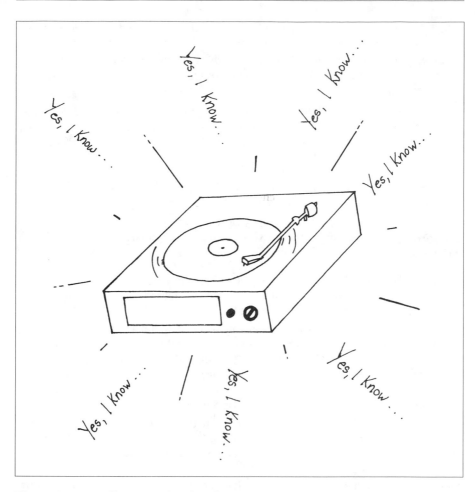

Figure A–2.   Broken record technique.

In assertiveness training this kind of compromise is called a *workable compromise*. It is a skill by which one works out an agreement with another person without either person losing or lessening his or her self-respect. The aim of the workable compromise is to resolve differences in position with another person.

Example:

ALICE: Betty, we agreed last month that we would each do our share of the cleaning of the apartment. For the last three weeks, I've done almost all of it myself. When are you going to do your part?

BETTY: Yes, I know you have been doing it, but I've been terribly busy. You know the band I play in is going into the competition next week. It's really important that I practice every night, and when I'm finished I'm too tired to be bothered with housework.

ALICE: I know it keeps you busy, but couldn't you do some of it?

BETTY: You know how important this competition is! I've got to put my practicing first. You aren't very busy are you?

ALICE: That's not the point. When I do all the housework, I feel like a doormat. It isn't fair to me. I think you should do your share.

BETTY: I know I should but I can't right now.

ALICE: I can see that the band practice is very important to you now, but I would like to work out a compromise. I'll continue to do the cleaning until the end of the month when your competition is finished. Then you can do the work next month, and I'll take it easy. How's that?

BETTY: That would be fine with me. Thanks for your help.

ALICE: That will suit me too. If I can count on you to do your share, I won't mind doing the extra work for the time being.

Exercise 13   Practice using the broken record technique and the workable compromise on the following examples:

1. *Broken record.* You are out shopping for a blouse. You have decided you want a blue one. The salesperson insists you choose a green blouse, saying, "You look much better in green. Take my word for it, get green."

2. *Workable compromise.* You feel you are overloaded at work and your boss asks you to take on the organization of the office Christmas party. You would enjoy doing this more than some of your other responsibilities, but you know your other duties will not get done properly.

3. *Broken record.* You are asked out on a date by a man you are not attracted to. He persists in trying to persuade you to date him.

4. *Workable compromise.* You accept an invitation to attend a party on Saturday night assuming you will have the use of the family car. On Friday, your son informs you he has made a date for Saturday night and needs the car.

Note: Make up other scenarios that are suitable to the needs and problems of your group members.

SESSION 6

Building Self-Respect

One of the ways we can build up our self-respect is to take time to identify our good qualities (Figure A–3).

Exercise 14   Write a list of ten qualities you like about yourself. Think of as many areas as you can—skills, abilities, talents, habits, characteristics, values, beliefs, appreciation of music, art, literature, nature. Begin each statement with, "I like the fact that I . . ." (e.g., "I like the fact that I am trying to become a more assertive person.") Keep your list handy and add to it when you think of other good qualities. Read it over whenever you feel discouraged about yourself.

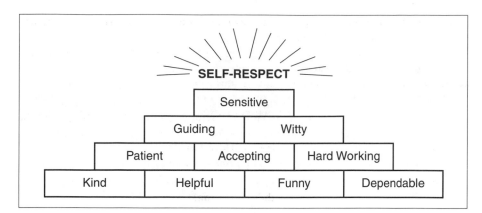

Figure A–3. Building self-respect.

Coping with Criticism

There are two kinds of criticism—factual and manipulative. In factual criticism, the critic is pointing out that we have made a mistake or that the critic objects to something in our behaviors. For example, the critic might say, "You are often late for work." In the second kind of criticism, the critic's goal is to manipulate or control someone by trying to make her or him change in some way. The criticism is not directed at the correction of a real fault or error, but at having the person do what the critic would like him or her to do; for example, "If you won't go to the movie with me, you are really inconsiderate."

Many of us have difficulty coping with errors we make in everyday life and the subsequent criticism we may receive. The criticism may cause us to feel anxious or guilty. We may become defensive, deny the truth in the criticism, attack, or try to please the critic. We can learn skills to help us cope with criticism in an assertive way.

Negative Assertion The skill used to deal with criticism of a real fault or error is called *negative assertion*. It involves:

1. Acknowledging our fault or error
2. Apologizing once
3. Acknowledging the effect of our action on the critic—that is, the critic's hurt or hostile feelings or the importance of our fault or error to him or her
4. Making amends, if possible

Example A:

MR. JONES: Look at this letter, Jean. We can't send it out. You spelled Mr. Smythe's name incorrectly.

JEAN: Oh, I see that I did. I'm sorry. I'll correct it immediately. I know Mr. Smythe is an important customer.

Example B:

MARY: Anne, you promised to drive me home from work yesterday and you didn't turn up. I was late getting home and then missed my appointment.

ANNE: I completely forgot! I'm sorry Mary. No wonder you're angry. Is there anything I can do to make it better?

Negative Inquiry   One skill used to deal with manipulative criticism is called *negative inquiry*. It involves asking clarifying questions in order to prompt the critic to be direct; for example, "What is it about what I'm doing that bothers you?" Having the issue clearly defined in an open manner increases the probability of finding a solution to the situation.

Example:

ANN: Joe, you shouldn't spend so much time working on that car every Saturday afternoon!

JOE: But I like to work on the car. What makes you think I spend too much time on it?

ANN: Well, you are always tired by the time you finish.

JOE: I don't understand. What is it about my getting tired that bothers you?

ANN: Well, when you are tired we never go out in the evening, and I like to go out on Saturday night.

Fogging   Another skill used to deal with manipulative or controlling criticism is called *fogging*. This skill is helpful when we are having difficulty saying what we really want to say because we are feeling angry, guilty, or anxious.

Fogging involves not resisting, but agreeing with:

1. The criticism, in principle
2. Any possible truth in the criticism
3. The odds that the criticism is true while still deciding yourself what your behavior will be

Example:

MOTHER: Mary, you really must make out a schedule for doing housework, and follow it! As it is, you are never caught up.

DAUGHTER: A schedule might help me to get caught up.

MOTHER: Following a schedule is the best way to manage a house.

DAUGHTER: You could be right, it may be the best way.

MOTHER: If you followed a schedule, you wouldn't have to do the laundry on Saturday.

DAUGHTER: You are probably right—I wouldn't have to do the laundry on Saturday if I followed a schedule.

MOTHER: And, you should give the children the same kind of schedule I used to make out for you.

DAUGHTER: Perhaps I should give the children schedules.

Note: Think of situations appropriate for your group members and have them suggest others where criticism has been an issue for them. Then, through role-playing, the members can practice the coping skills just presented to deal with the situations. Indeed, role-playing is especially useful in practicing assertive techniques and could be used very productively throughout all six sessions.

BOOKS USED IN THIS PROGRAM

Alberti, R. E., & Emmons, M. L. (1974). *Your perfect right; A guide to assertive behavior* (2d ed.). San Luis Obispo, CA: Impact.

Alberti, R. E., & Emmons, M. L. (1975). *Stand up, speak out, talk back!*. New York: Pocket Books.

Baer, J. (1976). *How to be an assertive (not aggressive) woman in life, in love, and on the job.* New York: New American Library.

Bower, S. A., & Bower, G. H. (1976). *Asserting yourself: A practical guide for positive change.* Boston: Addison-Wesley.

Fensterhein, H., & Baer, J. (1975). *Don't say yes when you want to say no; How assertiveness training can change your life.* New York: Dell Publishing.

YWCA (1989). *Discovering life skills, Volume V.* Toronto: YWCA.

YWCA (1991). *Discovering life skills, Volume VI.* Toronto: YWCA.

APPENDIX B

Small Group Program

Theme: Awareness of self

Sessions: Six

Recommendations:

For these problem areas:

1. Poor self-awareness
2. Lack of insight
3. Difficulty in recognizing and differentiating feelings
4. Difficulty expressing feelings
5. Social isolation

For clients who:

1. Have functional literacy level
2. Have verbal skills to participate in discussion
3. Are new to treatment

Objectives:

1. To provide opportunity to experience and express feelings, ideas, and opinions in a safe environment
2. To provide opportunity where giving and receiving feedback is encouraged among peers
3. To develop an understanding of oneself as an individual and in relation to others (i.e., how certain behaviors affect others)
4. To help individuals increase their awareness of others, the outside world, and what goes on around them
5. To sensitize the individual to the needs of others
6. To provide an environment for increasing social and self-esteem and confidence

Effective Aids:

1. Scissors and glue
2. Colored pencils, regular pencils
3. Newsprint/bristol board
4. Magazines
5. Paper bags

Activities:

Session 1: Magazine picture collage
Session 2: Drawing—How I see myself now. How I would like to see myself in the future.
Session 3: Life-line drawing
Session 4: The shield
Session 5: Where am I?
Session 6: Social atom

SESSION 1

Magazine Picture Collage

Materials and Equipment

1. Large round table and chairs or space to work in circle on the floor
2. Sheets of paper approximately 15″ × 20″—one for each person.
3. Scissors
4. Glue
5. Wide selection of magazines

Procedure The activity is introduced to the group as an exercise in which the members of the group will get to know each other through pictures. The leader should join in by making her or his own collage. Figure B–1 illustrates two types of collages: "Aspects of employment" and "Things related to travel." Instead of computer clip art shown here, group members would use pictures from magazines.

Group members are instructed to find pictures in magazines that illustrate the various aspects of their personality and life-style. They should look for pictures that show their interests, attitudes, likes, dislikes, characteristics, family, friends, job, feelings, ambitions, problems, and so on, (Remocker & Storch, 1979).

Group members could be given about fifteen minutes to look for and cut out the pictures, then perhaps another five minutes to glue them onto their piece of paper. It is best to clean up and set aside the magazines, so they will not be distractions during the remainder of the group.

Members are then asked to share their collages with the group. Suggest that they explain why they chose the different pictures and what each represents for them. Encourage members to inquire about pictures they do not understand and comment on those aspects they see as similar to their own. Monitor the time to be sure each member has an opportunity to share his or her collage.

Discussion Topics

How are members similar?
How are they different?
Are there any trends in the collages?

ASPECTS OF EMPLOYMENT

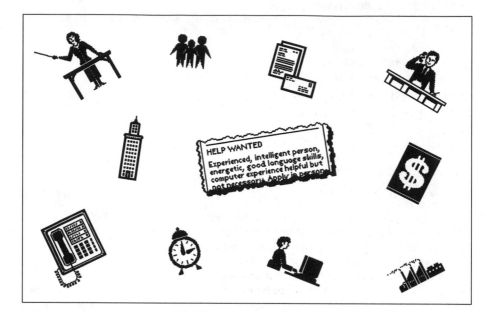

THINGS RELATED TO TRAVEL

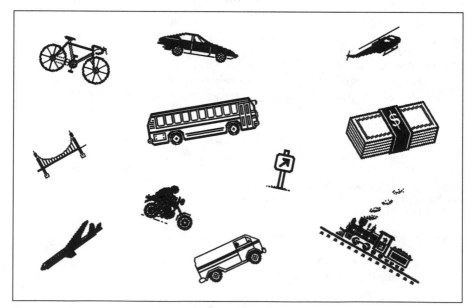

Figure B–1.   Collages: Employment and Travel.

Any aspects of themselves they would like to share but of which they were unable to find appropriate pictures?

What are the positives and negatives in the pictures?

SESSION 2

How I See Myself Now; How I Would Like to See Myself in the Future

Materials and Equipment

1. Large round table and chairs
2. White paper
3. Pencils with erasers
4. Felt pens

Procedure   While folding your piece of paper in half, invite the group members to do the same. Then instruct the members to draw, on the left side of their paper, pictures, diagrams, or symbols to portray how they see themselves today (see Figure B–2 for sample). Then, when finished with this, instruct them to draw, on the right side of the paper, how they would like to be in the future. Emphasize that artistic ability is not important in this exercise. Suggest that twenty minutes will probably be enough time to do both drawings. Be flexible and give a few more minutes if needed.

Ask the members to keep their papers folded and share only the pictures on the left side with the group first. When all have shared, encourage the members to find common parts or aspects of themselves. Then, ask members to share the picture(s) on the right side of their papers, showing how they would like to be.

Discussion Topics

What can I change?

How can I change?

The need to assume responsibility for making changes.

Fear of changing and fear of the future.

SESSION 3

Life-Line Drawing

Materials and Equipment

1. Large round table and chairs
2. White paper
3. Pencils with erasers
4. Colored pencils

Procedure   Ask members to position their papers lengthwise in front of them and then say something like the following:

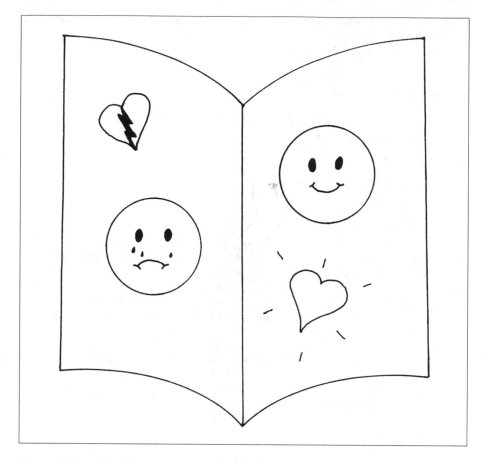

Figure B–2.   Symbolic depictions of self-perceptions.

Today we are going to draw our life-lines. We'll start at the left edge of our paper, and progressing across the paper to the right, we will draw pictures or symbols representing important—both sad and happy—events in our lives. Think back over your past and try to arrange the events in chronological order. So think of your childhood first and any significant things you remember about it and then your teen years, and so on.

Suggest members take fifteen to twenty minutes to draw their life-lines. When completed (Figure B–3 presents an example), invite members to share their drawings with the group. Encourage members to ask for explanations and to share similar experiences.

Discussion Topics

The most difficult period of your life.

The happiest time of your life.

Events where other people affect your life, and what you can do about it.

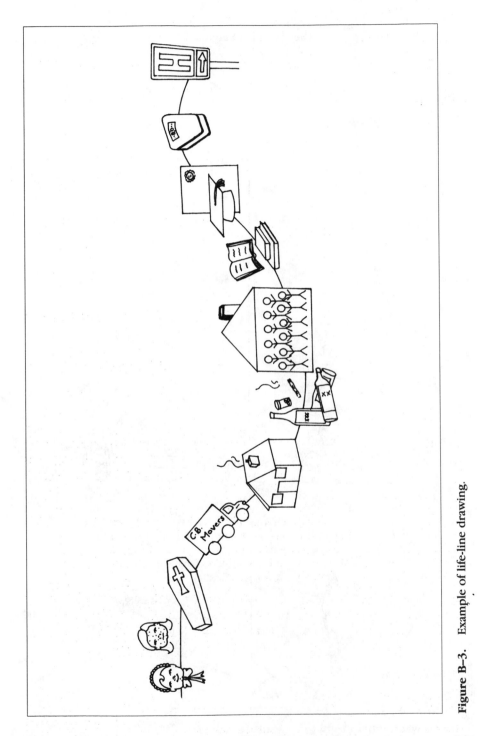

Figure B-3. Example of life-line drawing.

What precipitated periods when you felt in control of your life.

What precipitated periods where you felt helpless to control your life.

SESSION 4

The Shield

Materials and Equipment

1. Large round table and chairs
2. White paper
3. Pencil with erasers
4. Felt pens

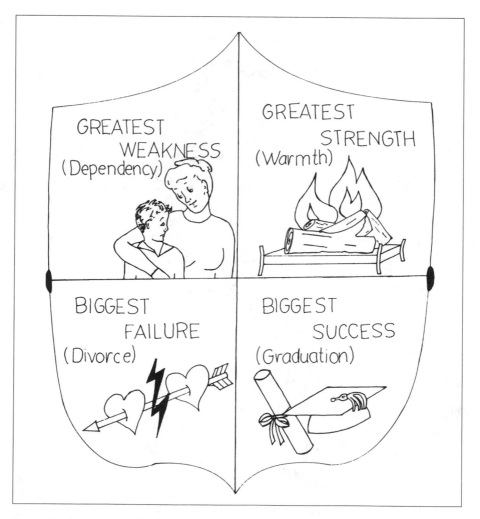

Figure B–4.   Sample shield.

Procedure   Ask members to place papers vertically in front of them. Explain:

Each of us has aspects of our lives that we are proud of and other aspects that we are not so proud of. We are going to present these in the form of a shield (*show drawing of a shield to indicate the shape and divisions*). So, draw a shield on your page and then divide it into four sections (*wait while members do this*). Now, in the four sections we are going to draw symbols or diagrams to represent aspects of ourselves. In the top left section, depict your greatest weakness; in the top right, your greatest strength; in the bottom left, the situation or event you consider to be your biggest failure; and in the bottom right, the situation or event you consider to be your biggest success.

Then, go on to give one or two examples,

For example, if I think my greatest weakness is depending on others, I might draw two figures with one leaning on the other, or if I feel my marriage is my biggest success, I might draw a heart or two hearts in the bottom right section. You will have fifteen to twenty minutes to complete your shield.

Figure B–4 shows a completed shield.

When members are ready, invite them to share their shields with the group. Suggest they share only one section at a time to ensure that each member will have one or more opportunities to share and to prevent important material from being overlooked or lost.

Discussion Topics

Can we use our strengths to help overcome our weaknesses?

How does failure make us feel, and how do we deal with it?

What about the usefulness of failure to motivate us to work toward success?

How can we have more successes?

SESSION 5

Where Am I?

Materials and Equipment

1. Straight back chairs
2. Signs with different attributes written on them such as assertiveness, patience, self-confidence, empathy, flexibility, humor.
3. Signs with "highest" written on one and "lowest" on the other.

Procedure   Explain to the group that the exercise is designed to help them begin to see themselves in relation to others. Ask all the group members to stand up and then say,

I'm going to move my chair out of the group for now and leave this space. On the chair to the left of the space I'll put the sign that says "highest" and on the chair over here to the right I'll put this sign that says "lowest." Then I'll put a sign on the floor in the middle of the circle with an attribute or personality trait written on it.

A depiction of what this would look like is shown in Figure B–5.

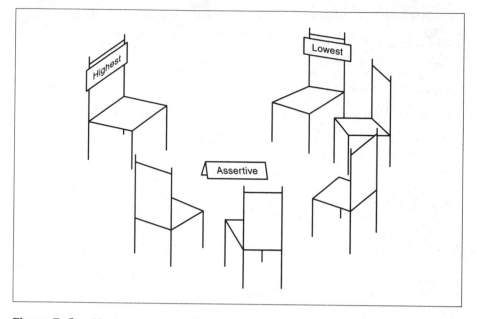

Figure B–5.   How assertive am I?

Think of this attribute as you progress around the circle from very little of it (the chair that says "lowest"), to a great deal of it (the chair that says "highest"). You are to select the chair that represents the degree of the attribute that you believe yourself to have. If someone else is in the chair or wants the same chair you want, then you have to try to negotiate a change with them by telling them why you believe you should have that particular position. If they believe you and think you are right, they will give up the position to you. If not, they will remain in the chair and you may have to try other negotiations. No pushing or shoving is allowed.

Judge when each exercise is finished by asking if all members are satisfied with their positions. Have members who are not satisfied try to negotiate for the positions they want. When the first exercise is finished, pull your chair into the space to rejoin the circle; ask members to share how they are feeling and how the exercise went for them.

When you feel the discussion on that attribute is exhausted, ask the members to put the next sign with a new attribute printed on it on the floor in the middle of the circle. Again, withdraw yourself and direct the members to repeat the exercise based on the new attribute.

Discussion Topics

Does the position that each member chose reflect their participation in the group?

Would you like more or less of the attribute?

Does the degree of this attribute that you have affect your life-style, work, or relationships?

SESSION 6

Social Atom

Materials and Equipment

1. Round table and chairs
2. Several pieces of paper per member
3. Pencils with erasers

Procedure   Explain that each of us exists within a network of collective social atoms. The number and content of collectives varies from person to person. Some collectives are more important than others. Also, the importance of the same collective may differ between individuals. (An example of what a collective of social atoms might look like is shown in Figure B–6.)

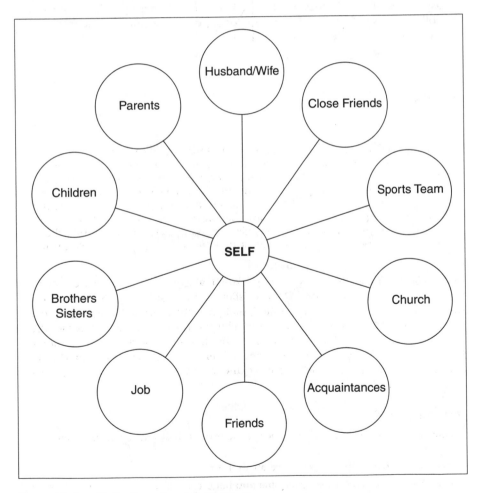

Figure B–6.   Collective of social atoms.

You might say to the group,

Take about five minutes to draw the network of Collective Social Atoms that make up your world. Now, on a second piece of paper redraw your network and place each collective in a position, relative to your "self," that represents the importance of that relationship to you. Do not consider whether the relationship is important to the other party, or whether it is a productive relationship. Only consider its significance to you. To be sure the relative importance is clear you might want to assign a number to each collective.

Member X's actual network is shown in Figure B–7.

Invite members to share and explain their networks to the group. If there is time left after each member has shared and the discussion seems complete, ask members to make another drawing of what would be an ideal network for them. Suggest they diagram the types of groups they would like to have plus names or fantasy names of people they would like included. Ask them to place and number the collectives as before to indicate the importance they would like the relationship to have. Member X's ideal network is shown in Figure B–8.

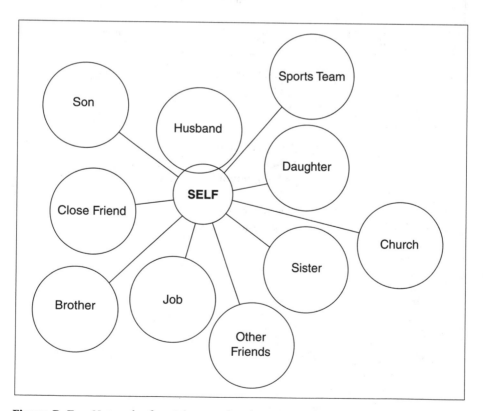

Figure B–7.   Network of social atoms for client X.

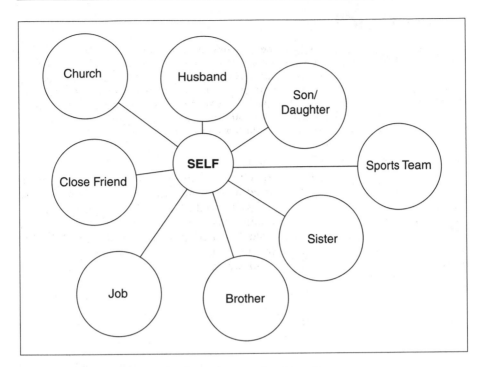

Figure B–8. Ideal network of social atoms for client X.

Discussion Topics

Discuss the number of collectives, the number of relationships within each, and the quality of the relationships.

Evaluate the collectives for vacancies, unfinished business, honest relationships, and those under strain.

Which collectives would you like to add, enlarge, or diminish?

Is it possible to make such changes, and how would you do it?

Index